The Paper Midwife

The Paper Midwife

A Guide to Responsible Homebirth

Ingrid and Paul Johnson

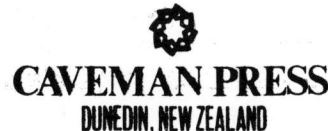

CAVEMAN PRESS
DUNEDIN, NEW ZEALAND

THE PAPER MIDWIFE... Copyright © by Ingrid Johnson and Paul Johnson, 1980. Sketches and Diagrams, © Jill Studd. All rights reserved. No part of this book may be used or reproduced in any manner whatsoever by any person or in any publication, or by any education or instructive institution, by means of photo-copy, stencilling, printing or reproduction on tape; audio and/or visual, without written permission except in the case of quotations embodied in critical articles and reviews. For further information address Caveman Publications Ltd., P.O. Box 1458, Dunedin, New Zealand.

Prepared and typeset by Mediaprint Services Ltd,
Dunedin, New Zealand,

Printed by Hedges & Bell Pty Ltd, Maryborough, Australia.

Layout and cover design by Trevor Reeves. Cover photograph by Paul Johnson.

ISBN 0 589 50279 4

Contents

CARING 7
WHO MAY NOT PREPARE FOR HOMEBIRTH 9
CHOOSING A MIDWIFE 12
NUTRITION IN PREGNANCY 14
EXERCISE DURING PREGNANCY 18
SEXUALITY DURING PREGNANCY 19
MEDICAL CARE 21
TO THE PREGNANT FATHER 23
ALTERNATIVES TO DRUGS 25
PREPARATION FOR LABOUR 29
    Nutritional
    Physical
    How to take Blood Pressure and
    Listen to the Fetal Heart
    Preparing the Birth Kit
    Photography at Birth
    Methods of Sterilisation
    How to Wash Up for Delivery
LABOUR AND DELIVERY 38
    Recognising the Onset of Labour
    Stages of Labour: First Stage
                         Transition
                         Second Stage
                         Delivery
                         Third Stage
    Management of Labour: Perineal support
                              APGAR assessment of newborn
                              First 10 minutes
                              Delivery of the placenta
    Labour and Delivery: Quick reference charts
MOTHERCARE 53
THE NEWBORN 56
CHILDREN AT BIRTH 61
BREASTFEEDING 63
IMMUNISATION AND CHILDHOOD ILLNESSES 69
PARENTING 72
APPENDIX I: *Problem Solving* 77
    During Pregnancy
    During Labour
    During Delivery
    After the Birth
APPENDIX II: *Supplementary Reading* 89

Caring

For whatever reason, Homebirth is returning, no longer as the fate of the underprivileged, but as a preferred alternative chosen by many people regardless of economic or social status. They are all people who care deeply about what happens to them and their newborn. There are some who approach birth at home with the post-hippie fatalism of "We'll just groove along with whatever happens, it's cool". Some, perhaps many, choose homebirth because they have seen the shining machinery of the delivery-room, its medicine men with their obscure rituals, and they are simply horrified, scared to death. There are also, within these young, colonial cultures, some extraordinary do-it-yourselfers who will pick up a book, such as this, and do it themselves.

Knowing why we do what we do can clarify our sense of direction and can help us get the most out of that event. This seems particularly pertinent to how we have babies. The Back-to-Nature urge is an excellent reason for questioning the new-age rituals to be found in the Delivery Room. Was there ever a really good reason for men to usurp that responsibility, or is it really the ultimate in chauvinism? Do the majority of hospital births need that bevy of nurses, anaesthetists, doctors, student doctors and whoever else wants to look in, or is it really that most births are, as Dr Gregory White tells the New York police, so straightforward that any normal eight year old could deliver the baby? (What an economic advantage if Maternity Wings dealt only with that 10% that warrant medical supervision.)

Is being scared of hospitals a good reason to avoid them? In the case of childbirth, a qualified 'yes'. The qualification is, if the mother is prepared to honestly assess her suitability for homebirth and then pursue the means for a sensible and safe alternative to the hospital. The problem with fear is that it inhibits birth. Mothers have dilated to seven or eight centimetres at home, gone into hospital and found that they have 'closed up' to two centimetres. Just frightened. It is not good enough to say "through education (or any other means) we must conquer that fear in women". The women most afraid of hospital births are those who have been through it once before. It seems as if medical and technological developments progressively eat away at our sense of self, our feeling of being an important, unique and competent person. Who is not afraid of giving up his, or her, free-will?

Being scared of hospitals and wanting something that seems more natural are widely felt and worthy sentiments, but an equally important consideration is the impact of that birth on the newborn. "I want the best for my child" no longer means a private room in an expensive private hospital. We wonder about children born depressed by drugs administered to the labouring mother; and about the mental scars left by forceps and various delivery routines; we wonder how the baby responds to the harsh theatre lights, the clattering sounds of stainless steel, and the antiseptic smell of the delivery room. We get desperately anxious when the baby, so thoroughly attached for nine months is suddenly whisked away for the hospital staff to wash, weigh, feed and dress — hell, who needs a mother! It's not at all difficult to imagine the enormous advantages most babies can enjoy in a warm, loving, touching, laughing and crying birth at home.

It is not merely the birth of the child, but is surely the Birth of the Family. Children who watch their brother or sister being born are special creatures, ones who understand the meaning of Family, who understand their own story. Fathers who break with their time-honoured roles as studs and breadwinners, who participate actively in the birth of their own children, seem to be unusually patient and caring; they are likely to laugh and play with their kids a bit more, and they also seem less inclined to put their jobs ahead of their family — a trait not appreciated in this workaholic world.

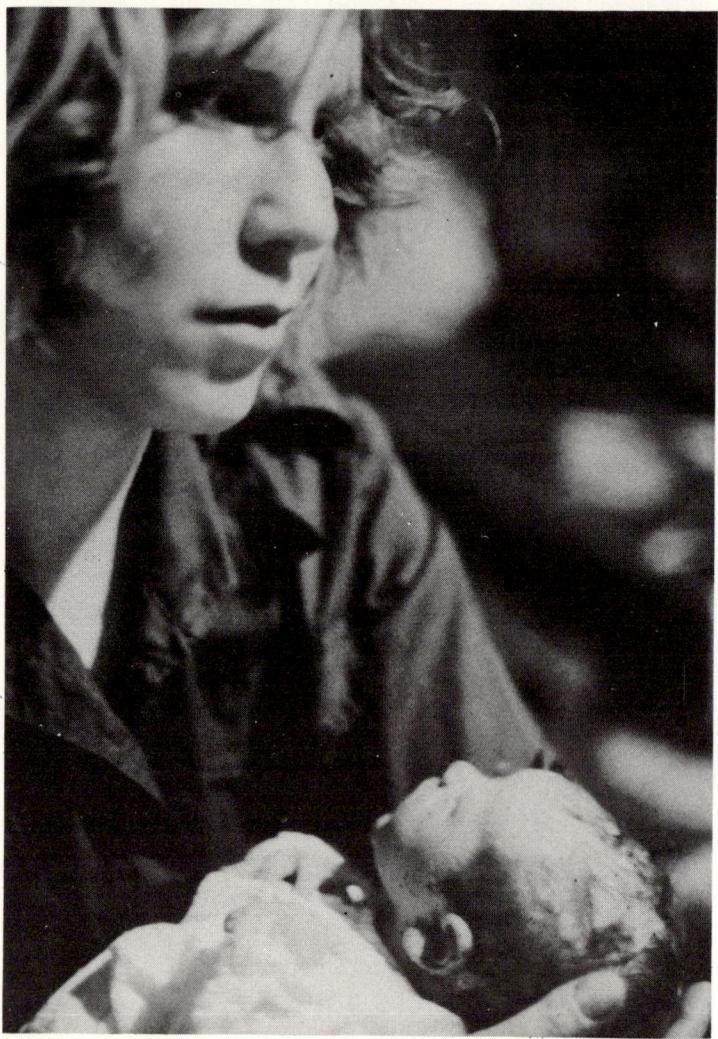

Ingrid exhausted after 36 hours 'on duty' as midwife

With growing support and the availability of information, a woman can gladly undertake the responsibility of preparing her mind and body, supplying all it needs to nourish her baby and herself, and to strengthen it for a reliable birth. Women are realising the inner strengths and sense of fulfilment that are gained from assuming responsibility for their pregnancy and birth; and the pleasure of incorporating this tremendous occasion into their life-style. Some of the most significant social change is born when a child is born at home. It is the proper place for loving, birthing, growing and dying.

Things most certainly are not what they used to be, thank goodness! Through scientific enquiry and experimentation, through various kinds of education, we are lucky enough to understand an extraordinary amount about our minds and bodies, and the healthy maintenance of both. Even better, we seem to be able to appreciate the importance of social health and discern the subtle ways that people, families and larger groups, can work to make or break each other. It is in this new age of informed concern that we can question the usefulness of our expensive and specialised technologies, designed for the needy few but imposed on the silent majority, and to be able to decide, for ourselves, what is best for us.

Medical information has always been held close to those who use its mystique for personal power and, perhaps, some economic advantage. Slowly, piece by piece, information on midwifery is becoming available to anyone, and even recent scientific studies and findings are surfacing for those who care to look. Despite the mystery, despite the aura that surrounds life's real miracle, Birth, we *can* pick up a book or two and intelligently decide "Should we do it at home?" and "How can we do it safely and lovingly?"

Who May Not Prepare For Homebirth

Unfortunately, not everyone who desires homebirth can feasibly plan for it. Certain important conditions must be met for the safety of both mother and child.

General requirements are:
1. Low-risk pregnancy
2. Emotional suitability
3. Physical and intellectual preparation
4. Suitable home environment and circumstances
5. Good general health and weight
6. Careful nutrition; no smoking, drugs, or alcohol
7. Regular prenatal checkups and a full knowledge of your medical picture
8. Intention to breastfeed

Conditions constituting a risk are:
1. If you have had Rheumatic Fever
2. Any abnormal heart condition
3. Diabetes
4. Toxaemia
5. A previous episode of abnormal bleeding
6. Rh or ABO incompatability

There are a host of other conditions which could cause a problem — teenage pregnancy, inadequate pelvis size, back problems, kidney disease, V.D., syphilis, contact with German measles .... Each woman must be individually assessed and advised as to whether her risk is great or small. Under certain conditions, a risk might not automatically eliminate a homebirth. Under competent doctor or midwife supervision, teenage mothers, overweight mothers, women with pelvic disproportion or Rh incompatibility have delivered safely at home. What is most important is a very, very careful evaluation of the risk and full knowledge of the possible consequences.

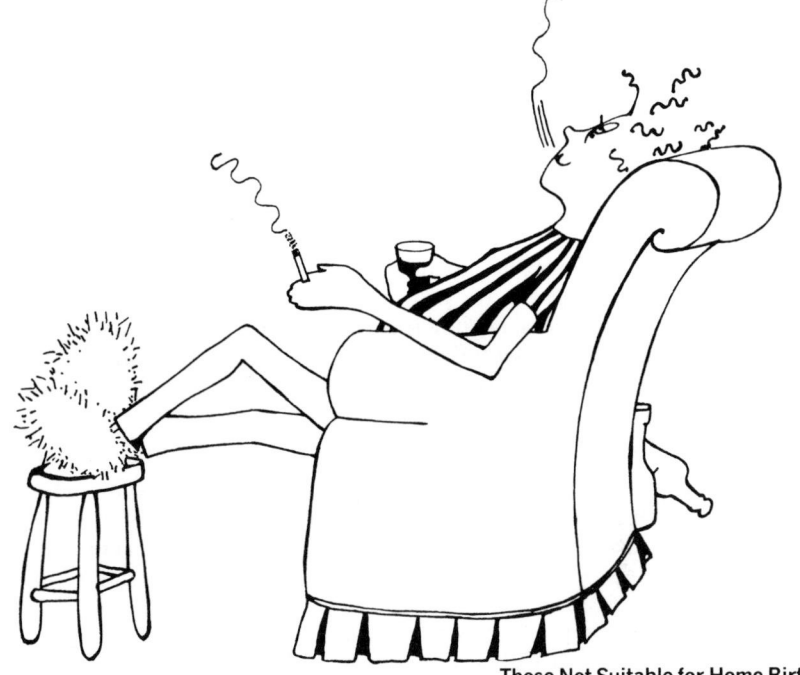
Those Not Suitable for Home Birth

Medical opinion of high-risk conditions is very rigid. If you have a known risk factor and believe it may be coped with at home, read Suzanne Arms' account of midwife Norman Casserley in her book "Immaculate Deception". This could be another valuable perspective on the problem. If you choose homebirth with a known risk, you must, however, also accept the absolute necessity of a competent, experienced birth attendant present for your delivery. Influencing this homebirth decision should be the proximity of a hospital. If there is not one close by, then homebirth is not a wise choice. It would be especially sensible to book in and familiarise yourself with a hospital where a suitable alternative birth is possible, to avoid delay and confusion should the hospital prove necessary. This could be considered a wise move by any prospective homebirth couple.

Do not consider homebirth if any previous birth has been by Caesarian section. There is always a risk that the uterus may rupture along the scar line; in many instances vaginal delivery is possible and preferable following a previous section, but it should always take place under medical supervision.

Do not consider homebirth if symptoms develop during pregnancy to suggest Placenta Previa; nor if the baby is in a Transverse Lie — that is, does not engage head or breech first in the pelvis, but lies instead slung across the pelvic outlet. Baby has to turn, be turned, or be delivered by Caesarian section.

A persistent breech can only be undertaken at home if you can find a doctor or midwife who is experienced in delivering a breech presentation naturally. It can be done, but it requires special knowledge and skills.

At least 80% of all births are normal and uncomplicated. Of the remaining number, several, under skilful management, will incur no problems. So for the majority, whether or not to have your baby at home is a question of circumstance and values, not safety or money.

Once you decide to prepare for homebirth, choose carefully the people you discuss your plans with. Talking about it is an important way of making evaluations, sorting out your ideas and fears, but discuss it with people who will be helpful. Many people react strangely to anything that is different. Some will feel it as a threat to, or criticism of themselves; they will have you constantly defending yourself, and offering only stubborn disapproval in return. You can spend too much time salvaging your own self-confidence if you shoulder other people's problems too. Valuable help will come from friends who respect your intelligence and capabilities, and who do not view your 'radical' ideas as a threat to their own lives. If you have friends who are strong, personally secure, and 'together', discussions with them will be helpful and thought provoking in a meaningful way regardless of whether they approve of homebirth or not. Do not waste energy talking about it indiscriminately; this is unnecessary, unhelpful, and in brief encounters it is hard to give the impression of deep caring and responsibility which should be associated with homebirth. While the movement is new and vulnerable, this point is important.

Reactions after the birth may be unexpected, varied and interesting. You must prepare yourselves to cope with the effects of your older child's experience of homebirth. After Matthew was born to very dear friends of ours, the older brother and sister were woken to share the good news. Four year old Sean, hands on hips, demanded to know, "Well, who delivered him?" When told his Daddy did, Sean let loose a huge grin and an all-consuming pride in his father. Since then he has been heard saying to his friends, "Who delivered your brother? MY DADDY delivered ours!" Other parents might not appreciate the challenge. At times, in the face of indignant parents, it may be hard to remain detached and allow your child to express his experience his way. The older the child, of course, the easier it will be to suggest social considerations in the name of peace!

The above-mentioned friends experienced rejection by long-standing friends after their homebirth. One of Matthew's grandmothers was an invaluable assistant at his birth; the other grandmother was so upset she hung-up the phone, and later said she didn't believe he could be normal after their doing it 'that way'. Was it for money? These reactions are not extreme or unusual; there will always be those who are appalled and those who admire and envy you. While hostile reactions from friends and loved ones is a hurtful shock, it is easier to handle opposition with a healthy babe-in-arms and the possession of a beautiful experience that no one can take away from you. Throughout, it is your own thread of self-confidence and flexibility that counts; don't let anyone turn it into a tightrope.

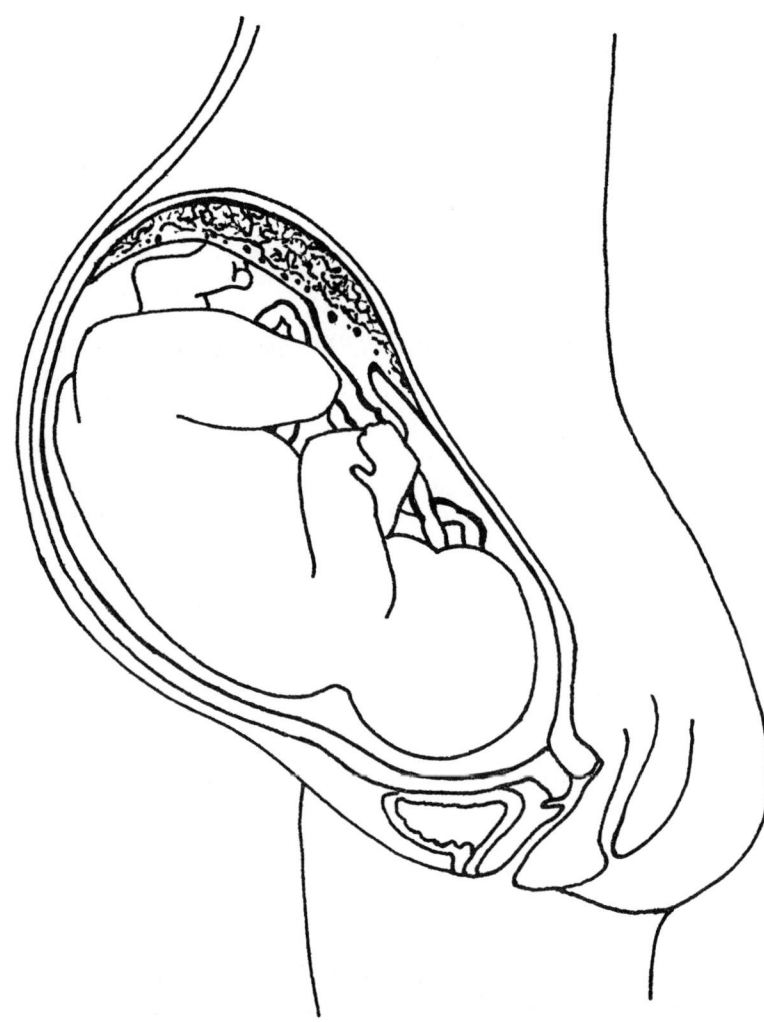

A Very
Pregnant Uterus

Choosing a Midwife

This manual endeavours to bring together information and sources of information to enable you to conduct a safe delivery at home, by yourselves if, like us, you have to. However, before finally deciding to do it alone, you should make every effort to find someone competent to help you.

If you are lucky enough to have a doctor even consider your proposition, talk with him and think about him at length before giving him the privilege of attending your birth. Some younger doctors may be more open to homebirth, but bear in mind that if he (or she) is a G.P., his experience in medical school has been very limited; lectures, doctor's rounds and about two months experience in his final two years of obstetrics and gynaecology. Has he ever witnessed a natural birth? An older doctor might bring with him a hospital atmosphere and its tensions and not fit in at all with your desire for an unhurried, unmedicated and naturally flowing birth. You are not doing your doctor an injustice by questioning his attitudes and values. If he can meet all your requirements and you, his, then take the chance. These are some basic question you need to ask him:

Will he be available to you day or night?
Will he be prepared to let a normal birth take its course without wanting to hurry it up or displaying impatience?
Will he remain in the background if the father wants to deliver the baby?
Can he agree not to interfere with the Third Stage of labour by not hurrying the birth of the placenta with various, dangerous, commonly used, hospital procedures - like painful abdominal massage and pulling on the cord, or even manual removal! He must be able to accept that while the majority of placentas are born within 15 to 20 minutes, a few may take two or more hours.
Will he accept other children being present? What complications does he consider will have a hospital outcome?
Will be agree to a gentle delivery for the baby's sake?
Has he ever delivered using perineal support instead of an episiotomy? If not, is he willing to learn how?
Will he read anything you may wish him to read to enhance his understanding of your needs?

If you live in an area serviced by midwives, your search will be much easier. Domiciliary midwives are available in some areas of the United Kingdom, Australia, and New Zealand. Health Department requirements vary, but if you plan a homebirth with a midwife attending, you can anticipate at least one, and preferably more, prenatal visits from her. She will be present throughout your labour and birth, and will visit your home frequently, even daily, during the two weeks that follow the birth. In North America, where lay midwives rather than nurse midwives attend homebirths, a great deal of time is spent on prenatal visits to allow the midwife and pregnant couple develop a friendship and rapport they consider essential to the atmosphere of birth. The more time you can spend getting to know your midwife the better, as there is no room in a normal labour and birth for personality clashes or professional domination. The ideal midwife will understand the kind of birth you want and make every reasonable attempt to fit into the atmosphere you create.

If you are absolutely unable to find an experienced assistant and want to go ahead with a birth at home on your own, you must accept that a great deal of learning is conditional to your making this a responsible decision. A midwifery text and related homebirth literature becomes mandatory. You must learn to hear and count the fetal heart and be familiar with its rhythm; you must study infant resuscitation methods and be able to respond instantly in an emergency. Most of all, you must become conversant with natural labour and all its normal variations. The following books, listed as recommended reading in Appendix II, have excellent birth reports: *Commonsense Childbirth*, *Spiritual Midwifery*, and the *Birth Book*.

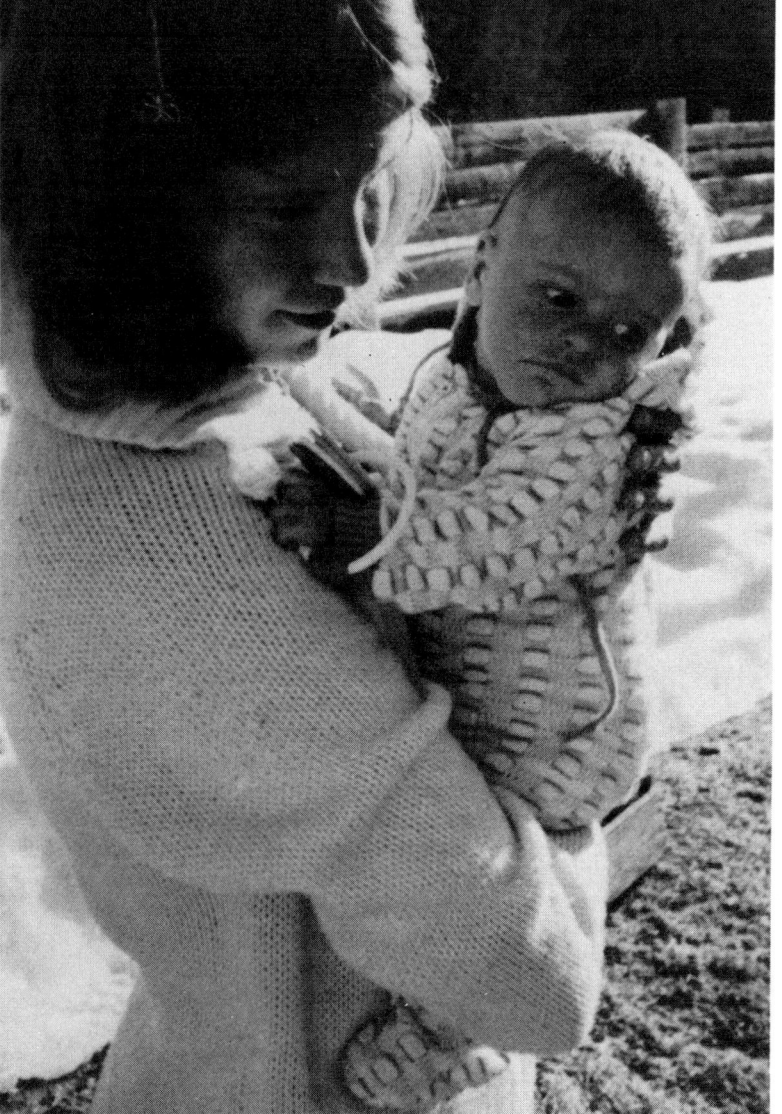

Nutrition in Pregnancy

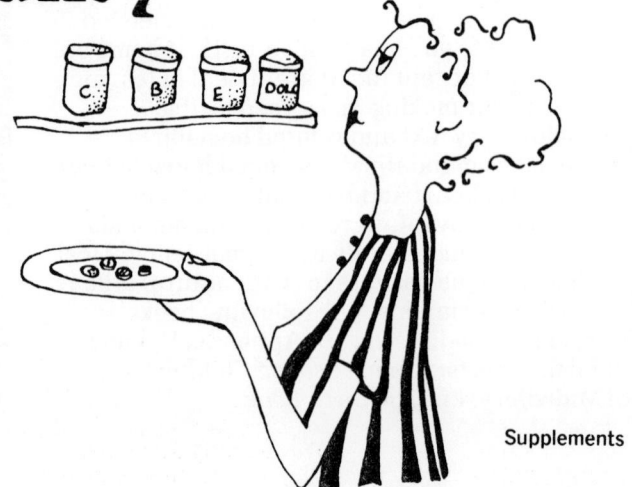
Supplements

This is one of the most important aspects of pregnancy because we can assume such control over it. Every cell in our body depends on the food, fluid and air we intake, and functions according to the quality of these elements. Our individual potential is determined by heredity, but whether or not that potential is fulfilled or starved depends on how we feed it, nutritionally no less than intellectually. Excellent nutrition is vitally important to the fetus who has no reserves. Certain deficiencies during intrauterine development can cause damage ranging from physical deformities, such as cleft palate and hare-lip, to improper development of vital organs including liver, kidneys, heart and brain. Similar irreversible damage may be the result of drugs taken during pregnancy. Damage incurred in all instances depends both what the foreign substance or deficiency is, and also the fetal stage of development (damage during the first three months can never be reversed, yet this is when a woman is least aware of the new life — a case for preparation before conception?) It is, too a myth that the fetus will get everything it needs from the mother's body regardless of her nutritional intake. This attitude is both selfish and risky. Inhaled smoke occupies valuable space in the bloodstream which should be occupied with oxygen-carrying bloodcells. So the fetus' oxygen supply is diminished at the same time its body is filled with chemicals. The air we breathe may not be too pure any more, but by understanding our nutritional requirements and the effects of unavoidable pollution, we can properly provide for our bodies and our babies.

BASIC PRINCIPLES OF NUTRITION

Protein is most important. It is the stuff from which muscles, blood, skin, hair, nails and internal organs are built. It is needed for the formation of hormones which control growth, metabolism and sexual development. It influences blood clotting, enzyme and antibody formation, and is also a source of energy. During pregnancy 75 - 90 grams of protein must be consumed daily. Meat, eggs, and dairy foods are sources of whole protein. Vegetarians must combine foods with full knowledge of their animo-acid content in order to get a substantial amount of complete protein in a meal. All women pregnant during summer must be especially aware of their protein intake, as at this time of year we tend to want lighter meals and salads instead of meals rich in protein, foods which tend to feel 'heavy' in the heat.

While high in protein, the diet should be moderate to low in carbohydrates and fats. These are important, but must be in proportion and of good quality. Using vegetable oils, whole grains, honey, black molasses, etc. and avoiding white flours, white rice, refined sugars, heavily processed and prepared foods, pop, and 'junk' foods, will provide a good balance of useful fat and carbohydrate. The foods to avoid provide only empty calories. Apart from providing some immediate, toxic energy, the body can only store them as fat. But the good sources of fat and carbohydrate provide us with important vitamins plus healthy energy and reserves.

In order to get the most out of food it should be fresh, eaten raw where possible, or cooked lightly, never overcooked. Many important vitamins are thrown away in vegetable water, so use as little water as possible and add it to gravies or sauces. Steamed vegetables retain the most vitamins.

Fluids should be water or fruit juices. It is important to cut down on, preferably avoid completely, coffee, tea, cocoa, and all Cola drinks, as they all contain caffeine. This noxious substance, caffeine, does affect the baby's heartrate, makes him agitated, and, as some studies indicate, may affect his birth weight.

Tap-water is not particularly pure if you are on town supply, but we can improve it. It is a valuable source of minerals, and studies have shown that there is less incidence of heart disease in hard-water areas, very likely due to the calcium and magnesium content. Chlorine is a gas and will readily evaporate from the water if it is lightly boiled or left to sit overnight. A pinch of ascorbic acid crystals (vitamin C) will neutralise the chlorine in a cup of water. (Chlorine is known to destroy vitamin E.)   Do not diet to lose weight during pregnancy. If your food intake is well balanced and of good quality foods, your weight gain will be right for you. The kind of weight gain to avoid is that resulting from empty calorie foods. It is at last being recognised that a substantial weight gain is healthy. It no longer seems as if a high weight gain predisposes toxaemia, so long as the weight is not from fluid retention. Remember too, that not all weight gained is fat; it breaks down as follows

Baby's birth weight	7½ lbs	3.4 kilograms
Placenta	2 lbs	.9 kilograms
Amniotic fluid	2 lbs	.9 kilograms
Increased uterus weight	2 lbs	.9 kilograms
Increased breast weight	½ lb	.23 kilograms
Increase blood volume	4 lbs	1.8 kilograms
Fat	9 lbs	4.1 kilograms
TOTAL:	27 lb	12.2 kilograms

So upwards of 20 or 25 lbs is both healthy and desirable. An underweight woman at conception may gain around 50 lbs during pregnancy. This gain tends to follow a pattern, where about 4½ lbs are gained during the first 20 weeks, and the rest gradually and consistently over the latter half of the pregnancy. Do not fast during pregnancy; the toxins released into the bloodstream present a danger to the baby.

SUPPLEMENTS

Most of us are dependent on store-bought, non-organic foods, city-treated water, and polluted air. We know that eggs and meat may be contaminated with hormones and chemicals, and we cannot assume that we get full nutritional value from any supermarket foods. For most of us, then, supplements are necessary to balance the deficiencies in our supermarket food, and also to counter the stress that assaults our bodies from polluted air, water, and food with harmful additives.

Diets not including meat need daily B_{12} and folic acid supplements. Folic acid deficiency is quite common in pregnant women, or women on (or recently off) the Pill. (See Chapter: *Medical Care*). Bran flakes, wheat flakes, cheeses, prunes, some yeast preparations and seafoods contain very small amounts of B .

Avoidable risks to the unborn child

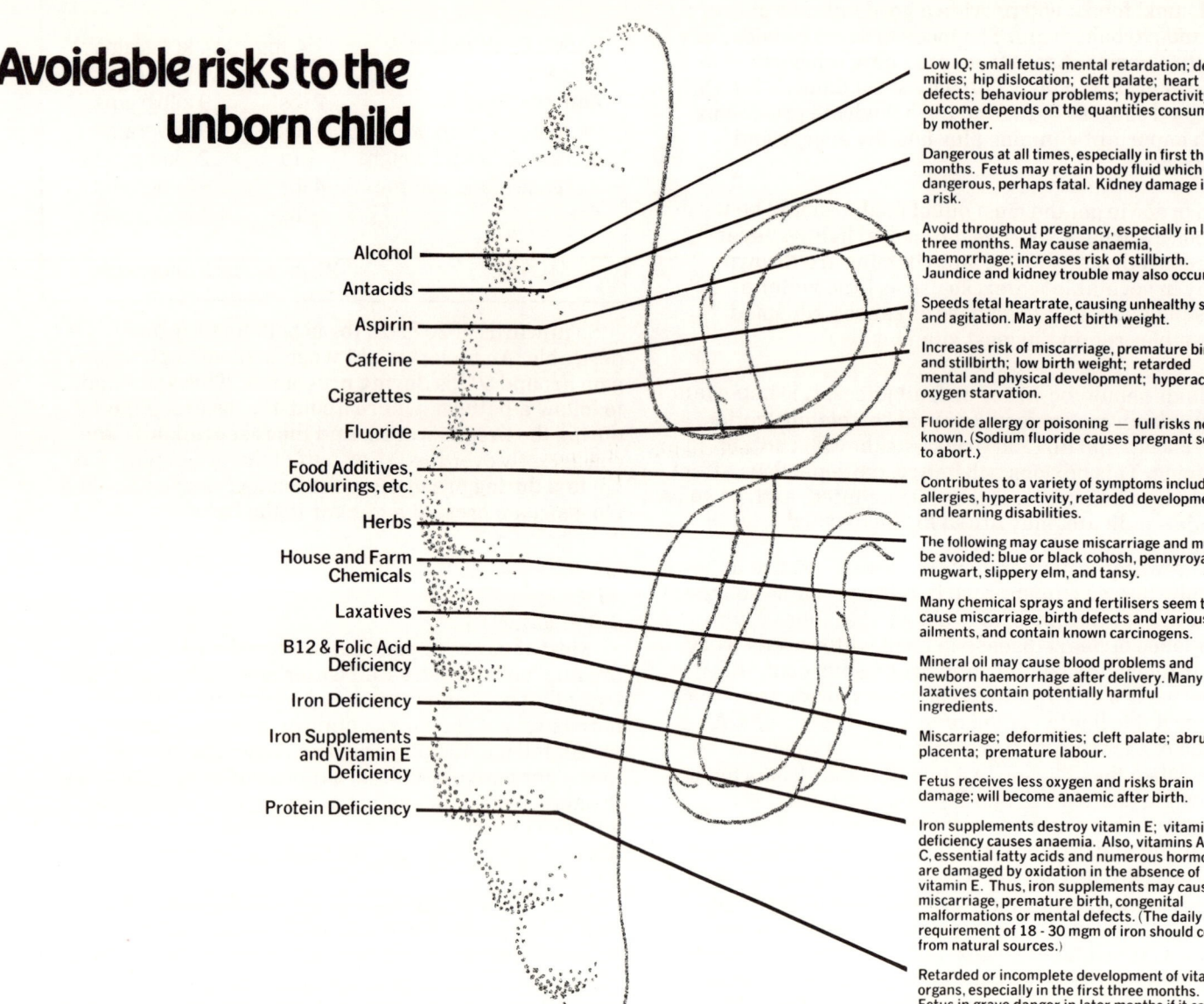

- Alcohol — Low IQ; small fetus; mental retardation; deformities; hip dislocation; cleft palate; heart defects; behaviour problems; hyperactivity.... outcome depends on the quantities consumed by mother.

- Antacids — Dangerous at all times, especially in first three months. Fetus may retain body fluid which is dangerous, perhaps fatal. Kidney damage is also a risk.

- Aspirin — Avoid throughout pregnancy, especially in last three months. May cause anaemia, haemorrhage; increases risk of stillbirth. Jaundice and kidney trouble may also occur.

- Caffeine — Speeds fetal heartrate, causing unhealthy stress and agitation. May affect birth weight.

- Cigarettes — Increases risk of miscarriage, premature birth and stillbirth; low birth weight; retarded mental and physical development; hyperactivity; oxygen starvation.

- Fluoride — Fluoride allergy or poisoning — full risks not yet known. (Sodium fluoride causes pregnant sows to abort.)

- Food Additives, Colourings, etc. — Contributes to a variety of symptoms including allergies, hyperactivity, retarded development, and learning disabilities.

- Herbs — The following may cause miscarriage and must be avoided: blue or black cohosh, pennyroyal, mugwart, slippery elm, and tansy.

- House and Farm Chemicals — Many chemical sprays and fertilisers seem to cause miscarriage, birth defects and various ailments, and contain known carcinogens.

- Laxatives — Mineral oil may cause blood problems and newborn haemorrhage after delivery. Many laxatives contain potentially harmful ingredients.

- B12 & Folic Acid Deficiency — Miscarriage; deformities; cleft palate; abruptio placenta; premature labour.

- Iron Deficiency — Fetus receives less oxygen and risks brain damage; will become anaemic after birth.

- Iron Supplements and Vitamin E Deficiency — Iron supplements destroy vitamin E; vitamin E deficiency causes anaemia. Also, vitamins A and C, essential fatty acids and numerous hormones are damaged by oxidation in the absence of vitamin E. Thus, iron supplements may cause miscarriage, premature birth, congenital malformations or mental defects. (The daily requirement of 18 - 30 mgm of iron should come from natural sources.)

- Protein Deficiency — Retarded or incomplete development of vital organs, especially in the first three months. Fetus in grave danger in later months if it causes maternal toxaemia.

Vitamin C is a highly talented organic substance. During pregnancy, along with vitamin E, it helps tissues to expand comfortably. In preparation for delivery, these two vitamins increase the elasticity of the perineal muscles. Vitamin C is a powerful detoxifier, breaking down toxins in the body from pollutants. Working with it in this task are vitamin E, calcium and zinc.

Calcium, magnesium and the B vitamins are essential to help the body cope with the stress of pregnancy, as well as being important for the developing fetus.

Doctors usually recommend prenatal multivitamin and mineral supplements. Synthetic preparations should be exchanged for natural source ones, as synthetics are not as effective, no matter how scientifically perfect. Also, synthetic vitamins cause side effects and overdose symptoms, whereas natural vitamins in the same quantities do not.

RECOMMENDATIONS

A one-a-day *Multimineral/vitamin* compound - natural source.

Folic acid, if you are not getting at least 1 mgm every day from your food. You can take up to 5 mgm per day.

Dolomite, which is calcium and magnesium in natural balance, to make up 2000 mgm of calcium and 800 mgm of magnesium a day. (Include food sources in your total).

Vitamin E, 200 IU daily. This will increase in preparation for labour, or for various other special needs during pregnancy. Get a natural source D-alpha tocopherol preparation; the addition of active, non-alpha tocopherols in some preparations is said to increase the vitamin E activity.

Vitamin C, at least 1000 mgm a day. The amount may be increased for special needs.

Iron supplements are largely wasted. The body absorbs iron from food sources much more effectively. A diet which includes regular quantities of liver, blackstrap molasses, brewers yeast, whole grains, yoghurt, and green vegetables, will provide the necessary iron and B vitamins.

Multivitamin preparations usually contain minimum amounts of vitamins A and D. It is wise to take extra - fish oil capsules are convenient - if necessary to make the total daily intake from food and supplements up to 25,000 IU vitamin A and 2000 IU of vitamin D.

A diet rich in green leafy vegetables will provide sufficient vitamin K. Yoghurt and some form of acidophilus - yoghurt tablet supplements - will supply the intestinal bacteria which produce vitamin K and the B vitamins in the body.

Additional nutritional requirements in preparation for labour are discussed in Chapter 6.

— Recommended Reading —

Davis, Adelle. Let's Have Healthy Children.
She includes calculation charts.

Nutrition Search Inc. Nutrition Almanac.
This is very informative, with detailed calculation charts.

— Bibliography —

"Smoking and the Fetus," Briefs. (Official Publication of the Maternity Centre Association). Jan. '77.

"Vitamin K Deficiencies in the Newborn", Briefs. Oct. '77.

Montague, Ashley, Life Before Birth
This has relevant chapters on diet, drugs, alcohol and smoking. (N.B. More recent studies give more serious views on the effects of alcohol than stated in this book).

"Perinatal Pharmacology". Birth & The Family Journal, Vol1, No.3.

"Drugs and the Fetus", Birth & The Family Journal, Vol 5. No.2.

"Folic Acid Deficiency Survey", Prevention, Sept. '78.

"Nutrition Against Pollution", Prevention, Aug. '78.

"Nutrition and Birth", Maternity Centre Assn. Booklet.
Summary of relevant reports; especially nutritional deprivation and its effects on the child; also weight gain in pregnancy.

Robe, Lucy Just So It's Healthy.
The effects of alcohol and specific drugs on pregnancy (she takes a rather narrow, 'medical' attitude to vitamins).

Rodale, J.I. Encyclopaedia For Healthy Living.

Exercise during Pregnancy

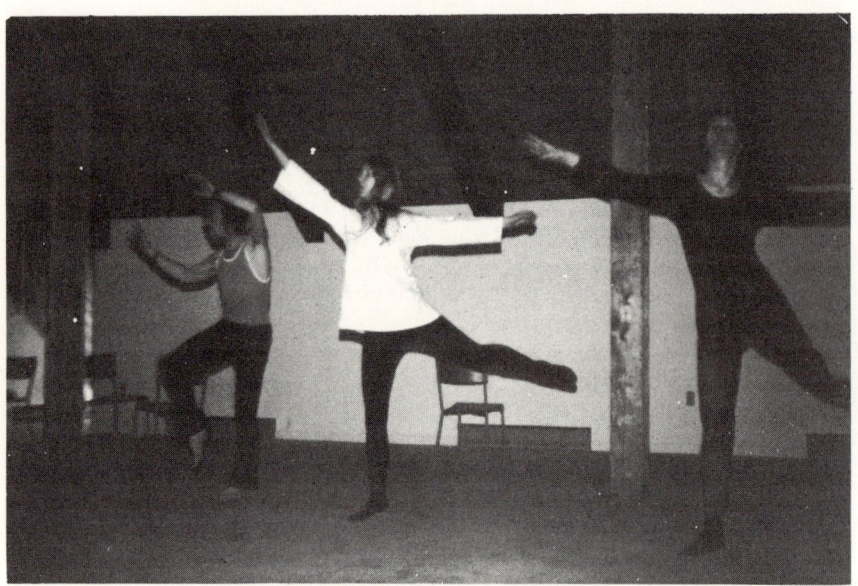

Maintain the activities you are accustomed to, dancing, yoga, swimming, with the one possible exception - horseriding. Modify them when you feel the need, according to how you feel. If you don't get much exercise, begin right away the habit of daily walks, and get involved with prenatal yoga (but avoid inverted positions in the last weeks when the baby may become engaged — there would be a risk of trapping and pinching the umbilical cord.).

Careful movement and good posture is important and attractive any time, but especially during pregnancy. You can do almost anything you want if you do it properly. When lifting, lift with your arms and thigh muscles, not your back; when going upstairs, take them gracefully, one at a time; roll on to your side and push yourself up with your arms when you get up from lying down; walk tall, pull yourself up through the top of your head — slumping exaggerates sway back, which causes headache, fatigue and general discomfort. Sitting in the tailor position, legs crossed and back curved forward, is a good counter position for the back, relieving the strain.

The amount of exercise you can handle may vary from day to day. Listen to your body and trust it. Don't pamper it; though pregnant, it is still in a natural condition and it needs exercise in a new, vital way. On the other hand don't ignore your pregnancy and push yourself to the limit. To work right up until you go into labour is not fair to yourself or the baby; extra consideration and rest is important.

Supple muscles may avoid some complications — such as some instances of breech presentation — and may help overcome others during delivery. It is never too early to begin exercising the pelvic floor muscles. Control over, and elasticity of these muscles makes a huge difference to delivery and recovery. A woman who has this control, and an attendant able to support the perineum during the birth can, between them, almost always avoid tearing.

If you travel while pregnant, be kind to yourself. If travelling by car, allow extra time for stretching your legs every hour or so to help your circulation. Lying on the seat on your left side is also good for your circulation. Don't neglect your bladder!

Flying over 5000ft in an unpressurised aircraft may place undue strain on the oxygen supply to your baby. Try to avoid travelling if you are prone to motion-sickness — most travel pills are not recommended during pregnancy.

— Recommended Reading —

Medvin, Jeannine.   Prenatal Yoga and Natural Birth
Bing, Elizabeth.   Moving Through Pregnancy
Dilfer, Carol.   Your Baby, Your Body

Sexuality during Pregnancy

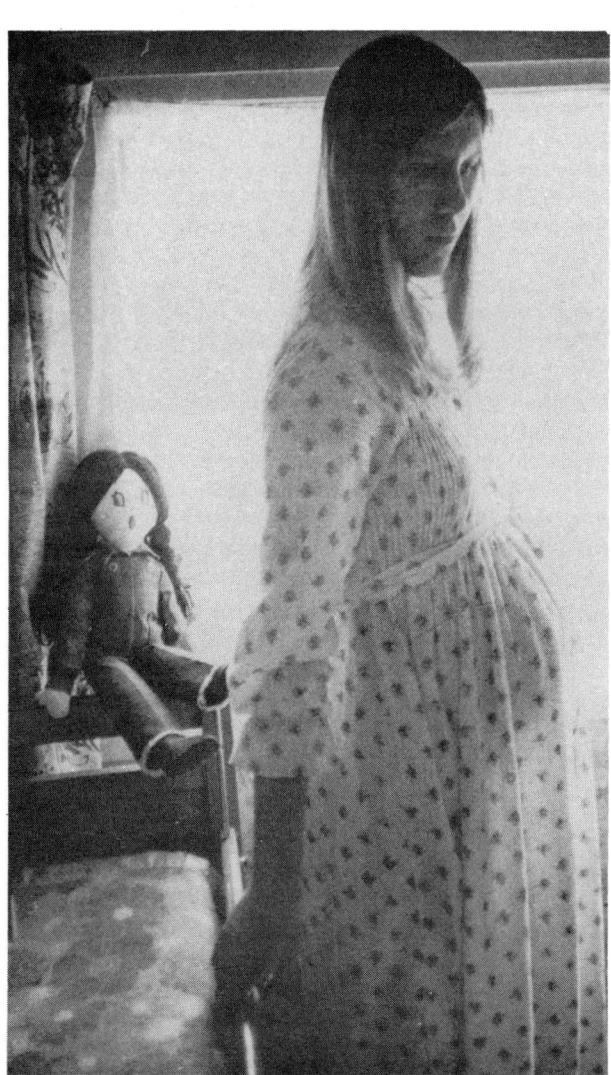

This topic has to take the award for the greatest number of myths obscuring it. Now there is, mercifully, a lot more reliable information emerging to put this into a healthier perspective.

Briefly, and assuming yours is a pregnancy uncomplicated by anything requiring individual evaluation, there are no reasons why sexual intercourse should not take place anytime you want. This is a time for being open, honest and especially sensitive to each other. Your limitations should be your own, and flexible — not rigid and someone else's. Normal desire varies in every woman, and in every man, and changes are to be expected during pregnancy.

In the last weeks of pregnancy, the challenges of a cumbersome body can be fun. It may also be a fine time for physical and spiritual closeness without the need for intercourse. Most doctors advise **against** it, but on the other hand we are realising that in **a** warm, together relationship, this physical closeness enhances the flow with which a woman drifts into labour. The Farm Midwives demonstrate how effectively loving caresses dispel tension and assist labour.

It is wise to avoid actual intercourse if premature rupture of the membranes occurs (about 10% of labours begin in this way). Otherwise the rule is to listen to yourself, trust your body and respect your own feelings.

Once the baby is born, the 'medical' rule of thumb is, again 'don't'. At the six week checkup the doctor will presumably give his permission. Doctors deal mostly with women who were not having Prepared Childbirth, and who will almost all have had large episiotomies, and be bottle feeding their babies — all factors leading to slow healing and recovery. Homebirth mothers rarely need episiotomies; any tears are usually small and heal swiftly. Breastfeeding hastens physical recovery. While it is not uncommon for bottle feeding mothers to have a postpartum vaginal discharge for four to six weeks, breastfeeding mothers usually find it is over in about two weeks. Again it is perhaps wise to abstain from actual intercourse as long as the discharge persists. Some women have ignored even this much advice and had no problems. It's really up to you.

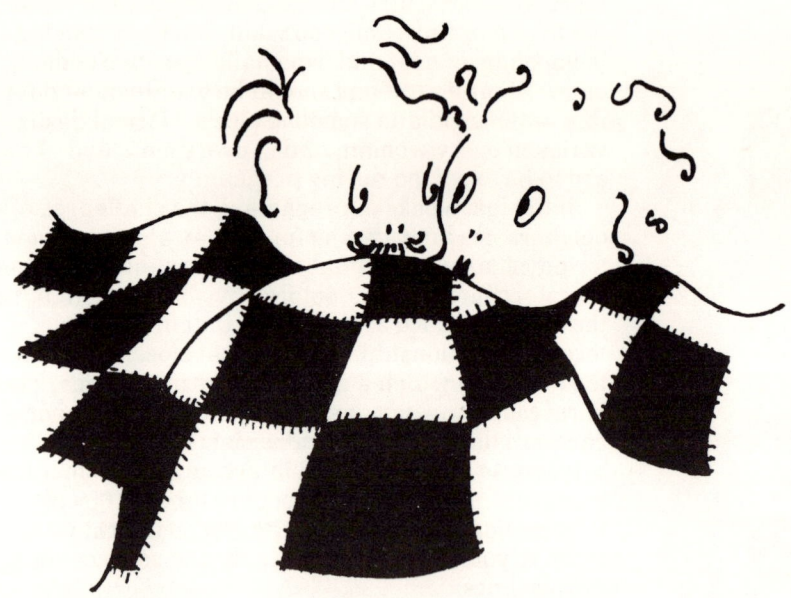

— Recommended Reading —

Bing, Elizabeth & Coleman, Libby.
    Making Love During Pregnancy.

Hazell, Lester   Commonsense Childbirth.

Kitzinger, Sheila   The Experience of Childbirth.

Lang, Raven   Birth Book

Medical Care

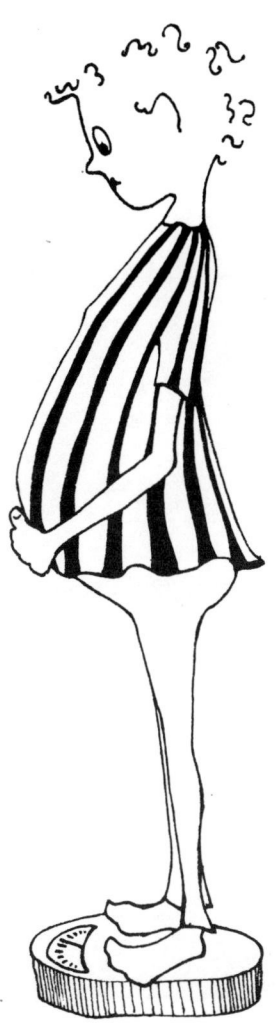

Medical prenatal care is one of your rights and a most important one. The doctor will assess you from a point of view you are less qualified to assess for yourself. He is continually updating your medical picture and the progress of your baby. He will pick up on things you may overlook and so good communication with him is important, as is an understanding of all he tells you.

He will do routine blood tests; you need to know your blood type to be aware of an ABO or Rh incompatibility. If you are Rh negative, your husband's blood must be typed; if he is Rh positive, you baby's blood type must be established by way of a cord-blood sample at birth, and you will require a Rhogam injection after the birth if the baby is Rh positive.

At each visit the doctor will:
- weigh you
- record your blood pressure
- test your urine
- palpate your abdomen
- listen to the baby's heartrate after he first hears it, at around the fifth month.

Doctors have individual ideas about ideal weight gains. If you eat only natural, nutritious foods, are not a compulsive eater, and limit your salt intake, you should not have to worry about your weight gain. Beware of anyone who tries to limit you to a meagre 20 lbs or less; great harm has been done in the past by such limitations. My own doctor panicked when I gained 25 lbs. I dutifully listened to him and went on to gain a total weight of 32 lbs, feeling wonderfully fit and happy about it. Some women, underweight at conception, have healthily gained 50 lbs during pregnancy.

Sudden, large weight gains and a rise in blood pressure may indicate toxaemia of pregnancy. Presence of albumen in the urine is a further symptom of this disease. The doctor will check your face, hands and feet for endema — fluid in the tissues — which also happens with toxaemia. This is why he'll usually ask "Are your rings tight?", the obvious discomfort if fingers swell.

Urine is also tested for the presence of sugar, as a kind of diabetes may develop during the added body-stress of pregnancy.

From palpating your abdomen, the doctor can tell whether the baby is the right size for the calculated age, and later, what position the baby has chosen to adopt; that is, whether the head or breech is presenting. A twin pregnancy may or may not be detected by palpation.

You need a doctor who will share his findings with you and will answer all your questions. You must be able to trust his sensitivity to your requirements should unexpected hospitalisation become necessary.

Where midwives are available, they work in close communication with your doctor or clinic.

If you decide to pursue homebirth where professional help is not available, you *must not* jeopardise your prenatal care by discussing your plans with your doctor if he might refuse to continue that care. Individual doctors differ greatly in their attitude to homebirth; shopping around for the most approachable doctor would be well worth your while. Even if he will not attend your birth at home, his assurance of help in an emergency is of tremendous value.

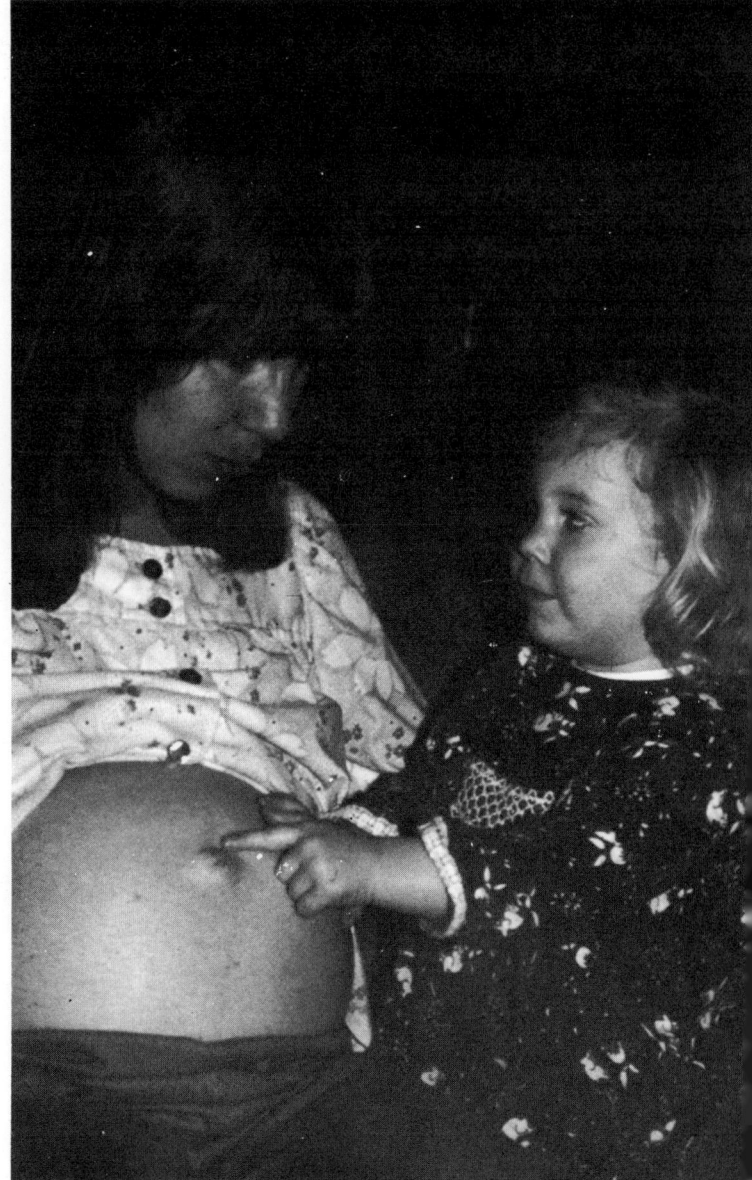

To the Pregnant Father

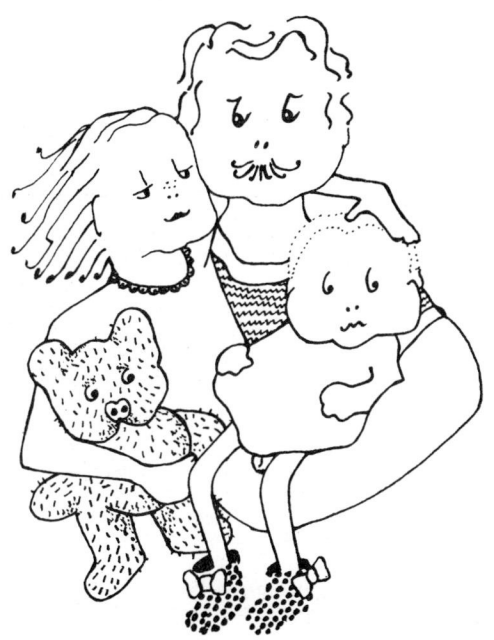

Many men feel unimportant because they are not biologically necessary for the birth. But although a birth will happen regardless of whether or not you are there, your supportive presence gives inestimable dimensions to the whole experience.

My two year old daughter was at her brother's birth, and it made her own birth story so real and comprehensible. The pride with which she says "My Daddy caught me" is as wonderful as the pride with which her father recalls the 'catching'. The bond between them is very special. Every man should be allowed to catch his own baby if he wants to, though not from outside pressure. Some doctors who attend homebirths are agreeable to remaining an observer during an uncomplicated delivery. I know of one doctor who allowed a father to deliver his child in a hospital labour room.

There is a lot written about the Father's role; some of it is sensitive, some rather chauvinistic, and much that is merely condescending. Search for your own values and never underestimate your importance and the ability that grows from intelligent research.

As I put all this information together I have in mind two people working together to benefit themselves and their baby. During the actual labour and birth the man and woman do have their own roles, but in the preparation, all knowledge, learning and practice should be shared because all the information is as important to you as it is to your woman.

It is necessary to mention here that a woman in labour becomes extremely single-minded; her whole body and mind is preoccupied with the job of giving birth. The attentions, encouragement, support and involvement of the husband and friends is absolutely essential, but she is unlikely to mention it at the time. It is usually some time afterwards that the man realises those back-rubs were a lifesaver, the fresh lemonade just what she needed, and his presence alone was utterly indispensible.

If you are planning a birth without professional help, some important role definitions must be worked out as part of your preparations. Some men who are going to deliver their babies get caught up and confused between the various roles of husband-father-coach-doctor. The husband and father roles integrate naturally, but the coach and the doctor are legacies from hospital-orientated conditioning. You are going to participate actively in an event that needs your love and full support. You are not exactly a coach (even in sports, the coach is not one of the players), neither are you a doctor. You are a concerned, responsible person who dares challenge the medical contention that *only* a doctor can perform the task that took him eight years to learn so little about.

A coach is somehow superior to his players; the doctor seems superior to his patient. The father-husband must avoid these power-plays by recognising the different kinds of energy and sensitivity that are needed at a birth. The woman in labour is an intensely physical and emotional creature, with no room for self evaluations or careful arguments — she is extending herself to offer the occasional thank-you. When, especially during transition, she asks if "everything is alright" or says, "I've changed my mind", the relative detachment of the husband is a valuable source of support with "everything is perfect, you are doing a magnificent job" or "I can see some dark curls". It seems most women display a good deal less anxiety than they feel, and these constant reassurances from the husband are truly deeply felt and appreciated. This kind of shared energy at the birth is, in fact, the birth of a greater unit — the birth of the family.

— Recommended Reading —

Hazell, Lester D. Commonsense Childbirth
(Husband as Coach).

Franks, Lynn. David, We're Pregnant!
(Humorous and sympathetic).

Alternatives to Drugs

This section provides information you may find useful, but use it at your own discretion. DO NOT gamble with any serious illness where doctors and modern medicines are the best resource. However, in many minor situations a little knowledge of alternatives can avoid unnecessary trips to the doctor and unnecessary medication. The following remedies are all natural, and may be taken without risk of clashing with other treatments you may be undergoing.

MORNING SICKNESS AND LETHARGY

There are several possible causes. It may be a deficiency of the B vitamins. For mild nausea, take a B complex tablet and extra vitamin B_1 to supply from 25mg to 100mg daily, and extra vitamin B_6 to supply 50mg daily. If you are vomiting, you may need up to 250mg of vitamin B_6; when the vomiting stops, reduce the amount.

There is a theory that nausea and vomiting of pregnancy could be due to some factor transferred to the mother from the placenta. In some cases, relief has been obtained by the combination of 25mg of vitamin C and 5mg of vitamin K daily.

If the condition is making it hard for you to eat properly, a low blood-sugar may add itself to the problem, causing lethargy and fatigue. Eating six nutritious snacks a day is a great idea; make sure they each include protein foods. Protein is most important for the baby's growth, and for the mother, and in two ways is relevant to morning sickness:

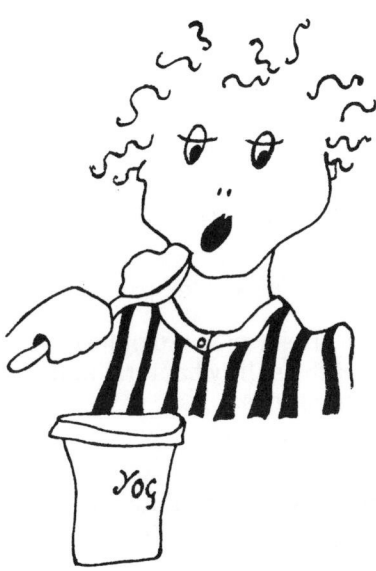

1. Protein foods raise the blood-sugar level slowly and steadily, and it is maintained for a prolonged length of time. A low blood-sugar does *not* mean you need to consume sugar; sugars and carbohydrates raise the blood-sugar very sharply, and after a brief interval it falls sharply again, and at no point will you feel any benefit.

2. Protein is composed of amino acids; one in particular, called Lysine, seems particularly pertinent to pregnancy. Lysine prevents anaemia, lassitude, chronic fatigue, high blood pressure and kidney complaints during pregnancy. Foods with significant Lysine content are: whole milk, whole eggs, liver, beef, fish, wheat germ, soybean meal, whole rice, whole corn, potatoes, brewer's yeast, and whole wheat.

INDIGESTION

Commercial alkalizers deplete hydrochloric acid, without which food is not fully digested. Consequently vitamin and mineral deficiencies may develop. Also, they are usually a form of sodium which is best avoided during pregnancy. (Sodium causes both the mother and baby to retain fluid — a potentially dangerous situation.) If indigestion is a persistent problem, examine your diet. It may not be providing a healthy acid-alkaline balance in the stomach. Raw radish relieves indigestion, as does papaya, fresh or juice. The latter contains papain, an invaluable aid to digestion. In one form or another, papaya is available from health stores.

CYSTITIS

Take Acidophilus Yoghurt, fresh or in tablet form. It provides the urinary tract with healthy bacteria and crowds out the disease-forming ones.

VAGINAL INFECTIONS

Acidophilus again, works as above. Acidophilus yoghurt can be applied directly into the vagina for prompt relief.

SWOLLEN HANDS AND FEET

Take vitamin B_6, 100mg daily.

BACKACHE

Check posture; sit often in the tailor position. Dolomite may help if it persists.

DIABETES

Sometimes sugar in the urine shows up during pregnancy. This becomes a medical problem and requires medical supervision. In addition, the following measures may prove beneficial: take 5 grains of garlic after each meal. Garlic lowers blood-sugar. Garlic is rich in potassium; in diabetes, acidosis robs the body of this It also contains zinc, which prolongs the usefulness of the body's insulin production. It contains manganese, which enables the body to remove sugar from the blood (onions, blueberries and nutritional yeast are rich in manganese). Garlic contains sulphur, which is found in pancreatic insulin. It also contains vitamin C, and assists in the vitamin C absorption from other foods (vitamin C acts like insulin - it helps metabolise carbohydrate in foods).

Honey should replace all other sugars. It contains Levulose, a sugar which is absorbed so slowly it does not 'shock' the system like other sugars.

Brewer's Yeast can help the pancreas produce insulin.

HAEMORRHOIDS

Take Rutin, 50mg three times a day. Vitamin E may help and can also be applied externally. Crushed cranberry poultices relieve pain promptly; and Lecithin 1200 can be applied externally.

HAY FEVER AND ALLERGIES

Eat honey; chew honeycomb to relieve sinus congestion. Comfrey tea with honey is soothing, relieving coughing and restlessness. Drink it at least four times a day during the hay-fever season.

Orange peels are antihistimines. Soak them in cider vinegar and bake, not quite to the candy stage, and keep them in the refrigerator; chew them as necessary.

ANAEMIA

Include in your daily diet; proetin, liver, garlic, kelp, vitamin B_{12} and vitamin C — in generous quantities. These items provide the body with usable iron and the means to absorb it.

CONSTIPATION

Check the fibre content of your diet. Include bran and wheat germ, garlic, raw honey and generous quantities of fruit on a regular basis. Do not use mineral oil or commercial laxatives; mineral oil coats the intestine preventing the absorption of vitamins and minerals and, in large doses, can cause kidney damage in your unborn child. Some laxatives do contain harmful ingredients that can be absorbed into your bloodstream and affect the baby's development. Furthermore, the use of laxatives disguises the fact that there is not enough fibre in the diet.

INFECTIONS

Garlic contains two potent, natural antibiotics — Alicin and Alliin — which are effective against a wide variety of bacteria, and sometimes more effective than penicillin. It is available in capsule form, and its antibiotic properties are effective for 10 hours after it is taken. If it is taken as soon as you are aware of a cold or any other problem coming on, it may halt the infection or considerably shorten its duration. Vitamin C taken with dolomite also has a kind of antibiotic action. It increases the number of white, infection-fighting blood-cells, and it boosts antibody production (Protein, vitamin A and vitamin B compex are very important in antibody production).

NOTE: Anyone taking antibiotics (medically prescribed) should increase their vitamin B intake, as B-forming bacteria are destroyed in the intestines along with the disease causing bacteria. Vitamin C is a detoxifier, and can decrease the side effects of many drugs. However, vitamin C is destroyed by most drugs, so it is wise to take 500mg of vitamin C every time you have to take a drug. Yoghurt or acidophilus culture should be taken with antibiotics to replace valuable intestinal bacteria.

PAIN RELIEF

Headache: Massage the tension spots; eat one tablespoon of honey and repeat an hour later if necessary (honey dilates the blood vessels); drink one teaspoon of honey and one teaspoon of cider vinegar in warm water; a steam inhalation of cider vinegar and boiling water.

Earache: Drops of liquid honey, or warm olive oil, or, vitamin E oil, or camomile tea directly into the ear are all very effective. Also drink the camomile tea. If the ear is infected, take garlic, vitamin C and dolomite tablets and continue the treatment for a few days beyond the relief of the symptoms.

Sore Throat: Treat as for infections. A clove of garlic kept in the mouth may relieve throat pain very quickly.

Toothache and Gum Pain: Rinse the mouth with Epsom salts in warm water; repeat at brief intervals until pain is relieved. Sage and cider vinegar applied directly relieves and cures gum ulcers.

VARICOSE VEINS

Vitamin E is needed, from upward of 400 I.U. daily, depending on the severity. (Diabetics need up to 3000 I.U. daily, with 2000mg of vitamin C.)

INSOMNIA

Soothing and relaxing teas are peppermint and camomile. Honey at bedtime is soothing and induces sleep; and garlic calms the nerves. Avoid all caffeine drinks — and that includes cocoa drinks and Colas too.

CRAMPS

If severe, increase vitamin E to 400 I.U. daily. Check your calcium and magnesium intake, and increase dolomite if necessary.

ASTHMA

Again, garlic is soothing and useful. Mullein tea, and comfrey tea, taken strong and daily, are both helpful — use honey for all sweetening. Red cranberry juice is a pleasant and helpful summer drink. Ensure that your vitamin E intake is from 100 to 200 I.U. daily.

— Resources —

Davis, Adele. Let's Have Healthy Children

Rodale, J.I.   Encyclopaedia for Healthy Living

de Baraclai Levy, Juliet.   Nature's Children

Robe, Lucy.   Just So It's Healthy.

Rodale Press   Prevention

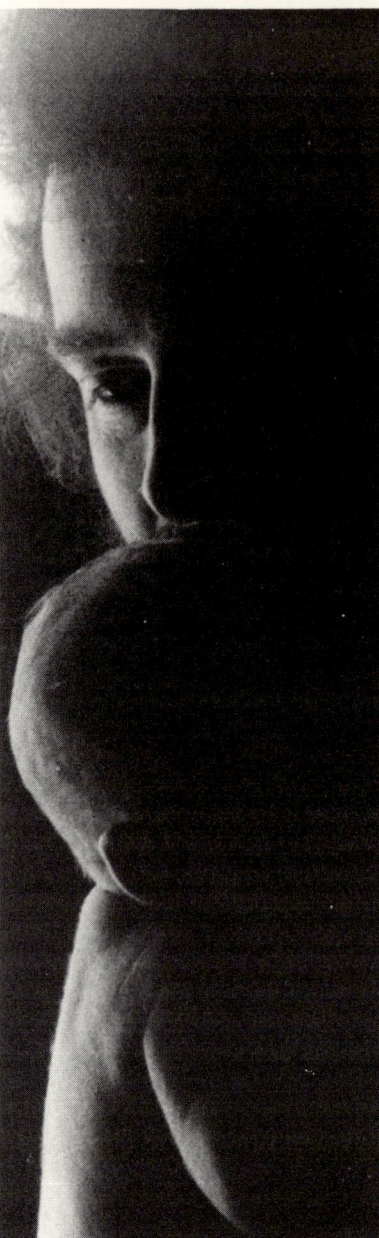

Paul and newborn Galen

Preparation for Labor

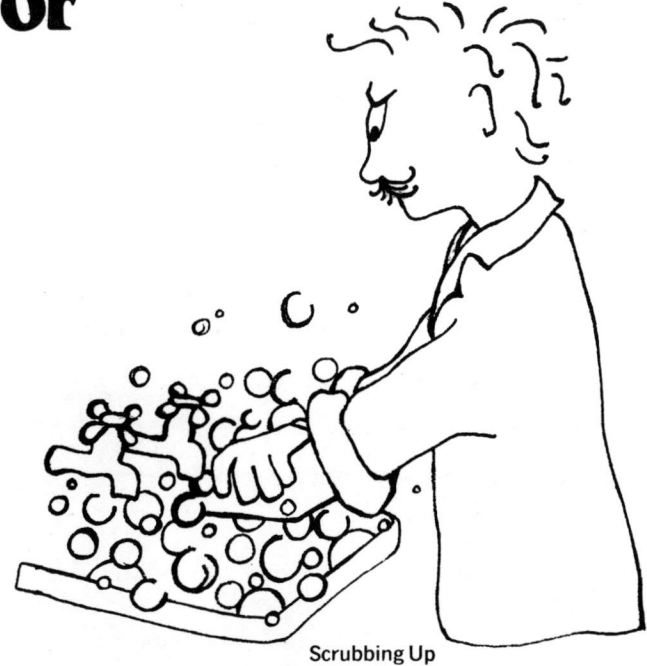
Scrubbing Up

NUTRITIONAL

About six weeks prior to your due date, implement the following recommendations, maintaining at the same time your high-protein, excellent quality diet.

Cut down on mucous-forming foods, like milk, to avoid mucous problems in the newborn.

Add a lecithin supplement to your daily diet. Lecithin aids the healthy development of the lungs, and assists in the easy establishment of breathing at birth.

Increase vitamin E to 400 I.U. or 600 I.U. daily for the following variety of reasons:
- it increases the expandibility and elasticity of tissues
- it strengthens muscles, making labour more effective
- it decreases any risk of blood-clotting (thrombosis) in the mother (a fairly common complication in women until recently, especially in those confined to bed for long periods)
- it decreases the risk of severe jaundice in the newborn by slowing down the destruction of excess red blood cells — (a normal occurrence, except that in the vitamin E deficient child, blood cells are broken down so rapidly that the body cannot excrete the end product (bilirubin) quickly enough, and it accumulates in the tissues causing jaundice); when severe, jaundice may do irreversible brain damage.

Vitamin E does not readily cross the placenta. Three hundred I.U. seems to be the minimum amount to take to benefit the baby.

Increase your intake of vitamin C as it is most important now to get the vaginal tissues really elastic and reduce the likelihood of tearing. Together, vitamins C and E reduce the possibility of haemorrage and anaemia. Generally, vitamin C reduces your susceptibility to infections at a time when you can well do without even the common cold. Recommendations on dosage vary considerably. However much you decide, it is most economical to add powdered vitamin C to juices.

Now is when Raspberry Leaf tea becomes effective as it helps the pelvic joints to loosen up in preparation for birth.

A note on herbal teas: there are several herbs of value during pregnancy, labour, birth, the post partum and lactation. If you know your herbs, use them sensibly. If you are not familiar with herbs, do not use teas indiscriminately. Herbs which cause bleeding, contractions or milk-suppression could do real damage if taken at the wrong time. Many commercial drug preparations are herbal based; though natural, herbs are not harmless.

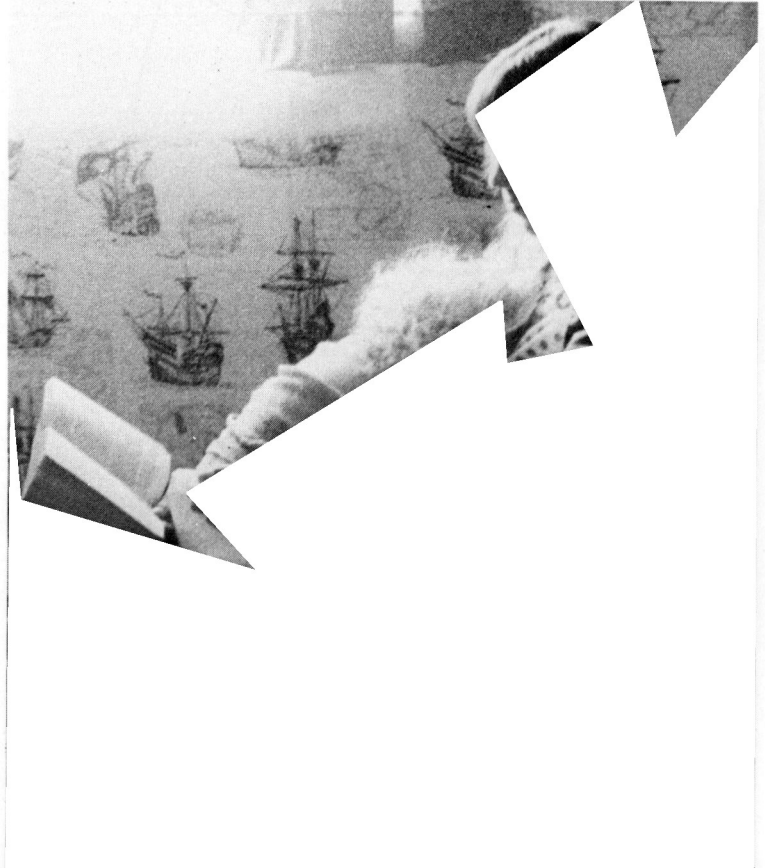

Awaiting the onset
of labour

PHYSICAL PREPARATION

Continue prenatal yoga, but concentrate now on exercises specifically for control during labour and delivery. Seven months seems to be an ideal time to begin relaxation exercises and breathing practice. If you begin much earlier, practice will drag; if you put if off much longer you risk having the baby arrive before you are comfortable with the techniques. Ideally, you'll go through a period of learning and perfecting the techniques, and baby will arrive while you are feeling confident, eager and ready to use your knowledge.

If you can attend classes run by Childbirth Education groups or midwives, do so, as it is much the easier way to learn. Otherwise, choose a method of Childbirth Preparation which appeals to you. Popular at present is the Lamaze technique which is certainly informative and effective for hospital births. The Lamaze relaxation and neuromuscular exercises are excellent training for body control during contractions, helping you to remain completely relaxed and free from distracting tensions. The Lamaze breathing techniques are designed to get the required amount of oxygen into your body, comfortably, and in a way that does not interfere with the action of the uterus. Once labour begins to progress strongly, the Lamaze technique employs "panting", rhythmical, high chest breathing. There is some criticism of this; the panting breath is classed as "unnatural", a kind of breathing we do not naturally adopt at any other time in our lives and which must be thoroughly learned and practiced for childbirth. However, it is obviously effective. A more serious criticism is the tendency to hyperventilate while panting; this could temporarily distress the baby causing acidosis from a shortage of oxygen.

When practiced properly, the Lamaze method is also used to relieve pain by distracting the mind from what is going on in the body. Many women, including myself, dislike this aspect of Lamaze. No-one preparing to give birth at home wishes to escape from the scene by becoming detached and insensitive to the experience. In hospital there are many interferences, and such an escape does become essential in order to maintain control; but at home this need does not exist.

Dr Robert Bradley, author of "Husband Coached Childbirth", has created his own preparation for childbirth techniques, based on Grantly Dick Read's findings. His attitude towards birth as a beautiful, natural, family event makes his book delightful to read and easy to work from. He is slightly condescending, and does not have the man's role in an entirely healthy perpsective, but has so much to offer of value, I can overlook this one annoying feature. The Bradley method does not employ chest breathing or disassociation techniques, and it is very effective. Many couples find it the most adaptable for homebirth.

Sheila Kitzinger, Britain's queen of Childbirth Preparation, is the author of several lovely books. Her psycho-sexual method approaches birth as a major experience within a life-cycle of awareness. She is very sensitive to family involvement and the importance of the place of birth. "The Experience of Childbirth" describes her method; "Giving Birth" describes parents emotions in childbirth and the effects on husband-wife and parent-child relationships.

Birth doesn't 'just happen'. Your body is going to do a lot of hard work for you, and what your body does becomes your experience, one you'll carry for a lifetime. What happens has a profound influence on everyone present for your birth. Be considerate to your body, as you would to anyone else who is going to work very hard. Your body IS you; it can only work as well as its needs are provided for. All good athletes prepare physically, emotionally amd nutritionally for athletic events. Success and personal fulfilment depend on preparation, and consideration of the body during the stress of unusual activity — particularly the nutritional and fluid requirements, and special breathing.

I care that when it comes to childbirth, 'natural' should not mean 'unprepared'. To drift through

How to Listen to the Fetal Heart

Where fetal heart will be best heard, depending on which side baby is lying.

• Mother's umbilicus.

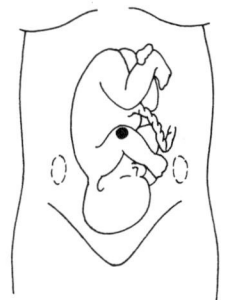

Fig.1 Posterior lie

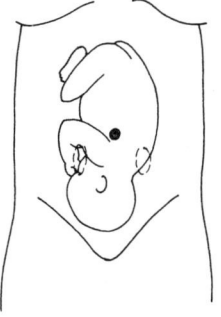

Fig.2 Anterior lie

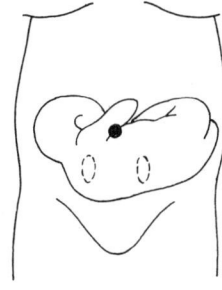

Fig.3 Transverse lie

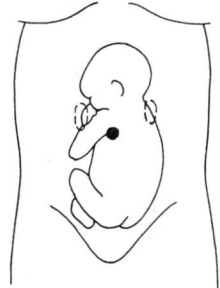

Fig.4 Breech

pregnancy, aiming to take labour and birth 'as it comes', is neither natural nor wise. Today, we have a wealth of knowledge and information which for previous generations did not exist, and to prepare thoroughly for birth is using our intelligence and obeying maternal instincts as nature herself designed. Unprepared-for birth may well incur the physician, with his tools and surgery, his drugs and anaesthetics, to conduct a birth that nature could never simulate, leaving in its wake only pain, fear, resentment, loss of all dignity, competence, and self-esteem.

Couples today seem more committed to the value of, if not necessity for, a shared and intimate, family experience. They prepare thoroughly for their birth regardless of where the baby is to be delivered; but to few, taking this precious event to hospital would be as unnatural as going there to make love.

The method of childbirth you choose should be used as a tool to increase your knowledge of what will happen in labour and how best your body can be assisted to cope most comfortably. It is the knowledge of what is happening that frees you from worry and tension, major causes of pain during labour.

Towards the end of the first stage of labour, during Transition, contractions become intense and difficult to handle (in most labours). During this brief period, at least, learned breathing techniques can make a huge difference to your ability to stay on top of it. Having some knowledge and resources to draw on at this time, is invaluable to the father and birth assistants to help the woman through a difficult time.

Giving birth at home leaves you free to prepare according to the method that appeals to you. You can act out as many variations on the theme as you like when the time comes, for you are not going to confuse hospital staff, invite their well-meaning corrections, or attract a crowd of curious spectators by doing so.

How you push during delivery is becoming a controversial issue. The Lamaze method teaches long, strong pushing with the woman holding her breath for prolonged periods. Some hospital classes teach you to push as if you were emptying your bowels. Vicki Walton recently pointed out to an appreciative audience, "It has been proven conclusively that babies are *not* born through the anus!"

Dr Roberto Caldeyro-Barcia, M.D., seems to be the authority on second stage labour; his findings alerted us to the dangers to the child of premature, artificial rupturing of the membranes. The gravest dangers to the child during the second stage of labour (expulsion and birth) are hypoxia and acidosis — oxygen deprivation. He contends that pushing techniques that urge the mother to bear down forcefully while holding her breath for prolonged times, are a major cause for the feared hypoxia. The child is born in better condition, both clinically and biochemically, if the mother is directed to push according to her physiological need and *without* holding her breath for an abnormally long time. He has found that five or six seconds is the general length of time for spontaneous efforts. Thus, during a single expulsive contraction, the mother would inhale several times as she bears down gently, compared to the two or three inhalations with forceful pushing as recommended in many techniques.

Second stage labour proceeds more slowly with this mild pushing, but the baby will be in much better shape. As Dr Barcia points out, this is a bonus for the perineum; it gets to stretch more slowly and lessens the likelihood of tearing, and in hospital births, episiotomies are greatly reduced.

HOW TO TAKE A BLOOD PRESSURE

The heart pumps blood through the arteries at a pressure high enough to send it through the smaller arteries and capilliaries, and back through the veins to the heart. The pressure is highest in the arteries, where it is usually measured; the unit of measurement is millimetres of mercury, and measured by an instrument called a sphygmomanometer. The heart muscle contracts, rests, then contracts again in a continuous rhythm. Pressure varies during the course of each heartbeat, the highest pressure occurring during the contraction of the heart when the blood is forced out of it (called Systole) and the lower pressure occurring during the relaxation of the heart muscle (Diastole). These two pressures are recorded when determining the blood pressure, the higher being written above or before the lower, for example, 120/80. The difference between the two pressures is usually about 40mm of mercury.

Procedure
1. The person whose blood pressure is to be recorded should be lying or sitting, one forearm extended and comfortably supported.
2. Wrap and fasten the cuff of the apparatus snugly and smoothly around the upper arm, keeping the elbow clear.
3. With your fingertips, feel for the pulse of the artery at the inner side of the bend of the elbow. This is where to place the stethoscope for listening.
4. Tighten the air-release screw on the rubber bulb; pump the bulb gently to inflate the cuff, until the pressure is slightly more than enough to shut off the sound of the pulse. The mercury will probably be at between 110-125mm at this point.
5. Listen carefully as you deflate the cuff. Watch the scale of numbers as the mercury descends; the point at which you first hear the pulse beat is the upper (systolic) pressure. As the air continues to escape, the pulse sounds become fainter and soon disappear. The point of their disappearance is the lower (diastolic) pressure.

Deflate the cuff fully and rest in between practices, or the arm will become very uncomfortable. Readings will vary slightly depending on the person's condition; i.e. whether she has been at rest, or very recently active, is lying or sitting, or tense, etc. But variations will be slight, and with a lot of practice her normal pressures will be apparent.

During pregnancy, a pressure which rises from a previously normal reading to 130 or 140/90 is dangerous, a possible sign of toxaemia. Following birth, a low blood pressure is a sign of shock, usually the result of unusual bleeding.

HOW TO LISTEN TO THE FETAL HEART

The following diagrams will show you where the fetal heart will be heard loudest, depending on the baby's position. If the baby is lying head down facing towards the mother's spine (anterior lie), it will be heard at this point — below and slightly to the side of the mother's navel (through the baby's upper back) on the right or left side.

If the baby's head is down but in a posterior lie, i.e. his spine against the mother's spine, it will be heard well over the mother's flanks, on either side. If the baby is breech, the heart will be heard above and to the side of the mother's navel.

With a stethoscope, a mother can listen to her baby, and most women enjoy this. For the husband, a stethoscope is not essential; with his ear pressed against her belly at the appropriate place, he will hear the fetal heart perhaps better than with a stethoscope which picks up all other 'plumbing' sounds as well. Most midwives will use a fetuscope, an instrument designed specifically for listening to fetal hearts.

GETTING A BIRTH KIT TOGETHER

The essential items you will need are:

Phisoderm or a similar skin cleanser for the birth attendant to use when he/she scrubs hands and arms ready to deliver.
Zephiran is a very convenient and useful preparation to use to clean the mother's perineum in preparation for birth. Use it in the same way after the birth. Zephiran solution will also serve to maintain the sterility of articles you boil up for the

delivery. A chemist might make up for you a 1 : 1000 solution; this strength is effective and safe on both skin and membrane. An alternative is to buy Zephiran concentrate and dilute it yourself using a gallon of sterile, distilled water (this requires care and precision).

When choosing your place to give birth, you must consider it from the point of view of comfort for yourself and convenience for the midwife. If you choose a bed, it must have a firm base. You may have to alter the dimensions, somehow, or use it sideways, to allow the midwife easy access. You may consider making a birth pad from a mattress or foam on the floor in a nice spot; you can use a wall, furniture, cushions and pillows for back support. Whatever you choose, get together some protection for the pad — newspapers, towels, sheets; or go the disposable way with incontinence pads or toddler's disposable diapers. Provide a table of suitable height beside the bed or birth pad on which sterile equipment can be placed.

Beyond this, you need to have on hand soft towels and receiving sheets for the baby.

The rest amounts to atmosphere, and this is your personal domain. People knit, play cards, listen to music, read poetry or philosophical books, chat, walk, do housework, sleep.... anything.... during labour. You will be free to do what you want, when you want and where you want to do it.

Ahead of time, do work out carefully who will be present during the birth. You need to know the people and be completely comfortable with them. Our needs vary in this respect. For some, a large group, a sharing of the experience is necessary; for others, it is a private moment in the lives of just a special few.

In an emergency, a husband can deliver a baby unassisted; in fact, a woman can deliver her own baby unassisted. But in a non-emergency event, a little more help will be appreciated. If a midwife is attending, the husband and one friend is about the minimum number; if the father plans to deliver alone, then two friends will be valuable to fetch, carry, and give

SUGGESTED BIRTH KIT

Alcohol

Surgical Gloves

Blunt-tip Scissors   preferably with about six-inch blades

Gauze Bandage   One inch wide, can be bought pre sterilised. This is excellent for tying the cord, as it holds a tight knot. Some sources recommend dental floss; but I feel that this could cut into the cord; and shoelaces - they can be awfully thick and hard to tie firmly.

Rubber Ear Syringe   From any chemist, is perfect for sucking mucous from the newborn mouth; it has a later use when the baby has his first headcold.

Sterile 3" x 3" Gauze Pads [or 4" x 4"]   These are available in chemists — the Bandaid section. Get plenty, to use to clean the perineum and also to use in the palm of your hand when supporting the perineum.

Umbilical Clamps   are essential if you have to cut the cord and clamp it quickly, but are difficult to locate in quantities of less than 100.

Bowls   A small one for the Zephiran solution, one for the instruments [although they can be left in the pot they are boiled in], and a large one to catch the placenta.

Flashlight

Clock or Watch with a second hand

Paper Bag for rubbish

Sanitary Pads

Some non-essential items to consider are:

Stethoscope and Blood Pressure Kit   Useful but not essential

Baby Bath   if the Le Boyer bath is intended. If you plan to use something portable, make sure it is still portable when full of water. Water temperature needs to be precise and so a water thermometer is a good idea.

encouragement and support. Everybody who attends the birth should feel useful. Another adult should be available if small children are to be present, to tend their needs while mum and dad are intently involved in the birth.

You will have to get a Birth Certificate and organise registration of the birth yourselves.

BIRTH PHOTOGRAPHY

Determine your photographic needs well in advance. A lot of deliberation can go into planning the lighting, borrowing the best camera, choosing the film and the photographer, if you want good photographs. You can't deliver the baby and photograph the event at the same time, and it is necessary to feel really at ease with the person behind the camera.

Any fast film (400 ASA colour slides or prints) may be 'pushed' to 800 or 1200 ASA without much loss of detail, and photo labs will compensate for this when developing the film for little extra cost. Whatever lighting is chosen, good picture quality comes from a uniform level of illumination — try to avoid heavy shadow areas. Subdued daylight will give excellent results, but since some births occur under tungsten light (incandescent light bulbs), a special filter is necessary to avoid orange-skinned people (fluorescent lights give skin a green tinge!) Electronic flash is sure to provide the right amount and 'colour' of light, but it seems like a violent intrusion into the gentle, warm atmosphere of a loving homebirth. A prefocused camera on a tripod is recommended for photographers who tend to get wet-eyed when babies are born.

Questions at this point seem to be, "Is this *all* we need?" "Is the birth safe without oxygen, a drug to contract the uterus, a blood pressure unit, or an I.V.?"

The blood pressure kit is up to you; you will only want it if the mother becomes feverish, ill, or displays otherwise alarming symptoms during labour, or else goes into shock following a haemorrhage. Either way, you'll need to get help; having her blood pressure does give you an added tool for evaluation, but from all other signs you'll recognise she needs help.

Do not be tempted to have oxygen on hand unless your birth is being attended by a person well qualified to use it, who brings it with him or her. Even in the hands of professionals, oxygen has been the cause of life-long damage, as a large percentage of permanently blind victims will testify. Oxygen is *not* a resuscitation measure; it might be used beneficially after a child has been resuscitated. Fill your body with vitamin E and rest assured that if your baby needs resuscitation, once he is breathing for himself he will promptly get on with living, for his body is not under the influence of drugs, anaesthesia or other depressing influences.

A midwife may carry some form of oxytocin, a drug used to contract the uterus to control bleeding. There are many measures (discussed elsewhere) to try first. If you do not have a qualified birth attendant, do not handle this drug yourself. Bleeding that resists all other measures needs medical attention. If you are stubborn, or live in an isolated area, refer to both 'Spiritual Midwifery, revised edition' and 'Pregnancy, Childbirth and the Newborn; a manual for rural midwives' for details on how to give intramuscular injections. It becomes your responsibility to understand all about the particular drug you intend to have on hand, the dosage, and the importance of a sterile needle and syringe.

Besides making you feel bedridden, victimised, a "case" to be pumped full of whatever the various doctors decide to slip into the tubing, the I.V. (intravenous drip) is now considered a danger because of its sugar content. The I.V. glucose replaces all the delectable tidbits you might naturally eat during labour, giving you a heap of glucose energy instead, which, hopefully, is not the kind of energy you are accustomed to and will probably make you feel sick and heady. We all know now that being confined to bed and uncomfortable prolongs labour, that drugs and lying on your back can depress and distress the baby. Now studies are finding that brain damage from a shortage of oxygen during birth is directly related to the amount of glucose in the baby's brain at the time; the more glucose, the greater the need for oxygen. This undoubtedly helps to account for the huge number of children today with brain damage ranging from minimal to maximal. Apart from the dangers, these accessories would change the atmosphere in your home to little better than a hospital setting.

STERILISING THE EQUIPMENT

You can sterilise linen ahead of time. Wrap the items into several small packages wrapped in strong brown paper and seal then well. List the contents of each package to ease later identification.

Bake them in the oven at 120°C for one hour. Have a pan of water in there too, to prevent scorching. Date the packages and resterilise them every five days until they are used.

A roll of sterilised paper towels is useful in lots of ways — if you separate them first and do them in packs of 12. They are very useful for the mother to use for cleaning her bottom in the days after the birth.

If you want a sterile sheet, or cloths in a hurry, iron clean cotton ones with a hot iron. This gets things super-clean.

Rubber and metal items are to be boiled during labour. Stand a pair of kitchen tongs in the saucepan while things are boiling as this makes it easier to

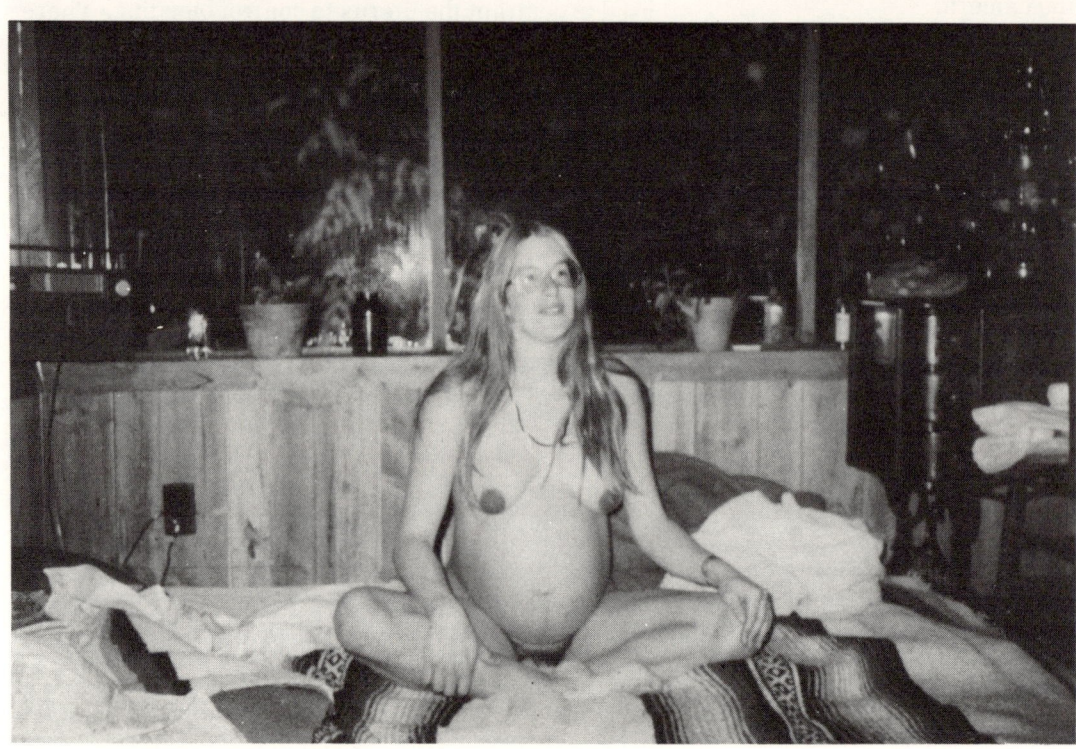

Laurie in early labour

handle everything and keep it sterile while transferring it to the birth place.

Items which must be sterilised:

- Scissors
- Rubber suction Syringe
- Umbilical Clamps
- Cord ties or Gauze strips
- Gauze squares
- Gloves for internal examinations

The gauze squares and one inch bandage can be purchased pre-sterilised from any chemist. Do not open the packages and you won't have to resterilise them. Cord clamps purchased loose will have to be sterilised with the other things, or you might find them in pre-sterilised packages too.

Linen should be sterilised if you are not giving birth in your own, established, bacteriological environment; or if your quarters are perhaps temporary and hard to keep clean; or if there are any animals around; or in any other situation where cleanliness is questionable. It is a good idea to have sterile linen anyway, although it should not be considered an essential piece of equipment in a sudden, unexpected birth.

While persons attending the birth need not be sterilised, their personal cleanliness is a matter of concern; no-one with any kind of infection may be present.

HOW TO WASH UP FOR DELIVERY

When a fair bit of the baby's head can be seen (or when the woman begins pushing if labour has gone fast; or if the woman has a speedy reputation) it is time for the father, or whoever else has the privilege to deliver the baby, to wash up.

Under running water if possible, wash up to your elbows with soap, lathering well. Scrub nails with a brush (nails must be recently cut short). Rinse, then scrub and lather up to the elbows again, using Phisoderm this time. Take your time, do it well. Rinse, and dry yourself with a very clean towel. From now on, just devote yourself to perineal massage and guiding the birth — other people can do the fetching and carrying.

Gloves are not necessary for the birth, just for internal examinations. An important exception would be if the person delivering had an infected scratch or sore on his or her hand.

Labour and Delivery

Learning about labour is important; most mothers I talk with say they wish they had known more. To learn more about it ahead of the experience is difficult, just as it is almost impossible to learn 'parenting' before the children are born. Before I ever gave birth, I had enough obstetrical knowledge to pass exam papers and to deliver babies as a nurse. But after our first birth I was amazed at how different the actual experience was and at how deepened my understanding became. Knowing all you can possibly learn about labour gives you the security of being able to figure out what is going on when the time comes. This, and the knowledge of the broad range of variations in normal labour will save unnecessary worry and confusion. It is a great advantage to have a midwife with you throughout the event to explain your progress; the baby is on a unique trip and it is fun to understand always where he's at. When labour commences he is only a few inches from his destination; why it can take him several hours to get there is indeed an interesting story.

When labour begins, the baby's head becomes engaged (if it is not already) in the lower part of the bony pelvis. With first babies, the engagement of the head takes place any time in the last four weeks of pregnancy; with subsequent pregnancies, it might not occur until labour begins. This process is also known as 'lightening' because the dropping of the baby's head into the pelvis considerably relieves the pressure in the upper abdomen. As labour progresses and contractions press the baby's head through the enlarging cervix, the head descends deeper into the pelvis.

The pelvic bones are held solidly together by ligaments. During pregnancy the joints loosen up and spread slightly apart to increase space for the passage of the baby. As the baby's head passes through the pelvis, the skull bones mould (overlap), and this mutal flexibility accomplishes the easy vaginal delivery of most babies.

The 'pelvic floor' is a sturdy sling of muscles which separates the pelvic cavity from the perineal area

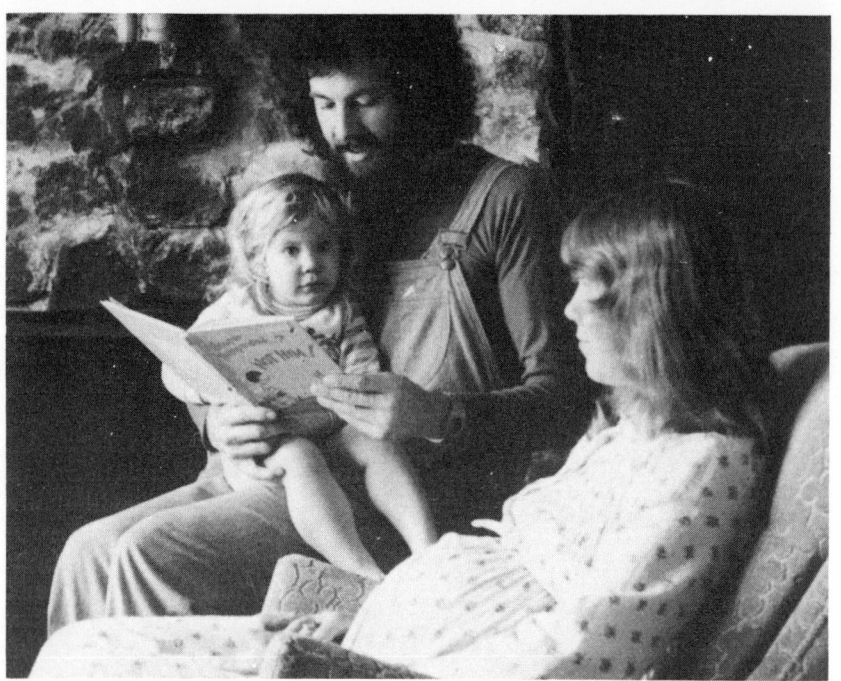

Ingrid in established labour

below. These muscles, which surround the urethra, the vagina and the rectum, are responsible for the control we have over urination and emptying our bowels. During late pregnancy, hormones cause these muscles to become very elastic, and relaxed enough to allow the birth of a full term baby.

The perineum is the external area between the woman's anus and her vulva. This is composed of both muscle and connective tissue, and is also capable of great distension to allow the birth of the baby.

The uterus is a hollow, muscular organ, the size and shape of a small pear when non-pregnant. Its remarkable ability to expand is obvious. Its outlet, the cervix, is like a bottleneck, one-third the size of the non-pregnant uterus, and up to 1½ inches thick. During pregnancy, while the uterus expands, the cervix remains thick and firm, plugged solidly with protective mucous; then as labour approaches, it softens and thins and becomes able to be effaced and drawn wide open. The cervix leads the way into the birth canal (vagina) which is lined with multifolded membrane and is greatly stretchable. The birth canal is about 7 - 10cm long.

Braxton-Hicks contractions are normal, muscle-toning actions of the uterus and are felt quite distinctly in late pregnancy as painless, tight sensations.

When labour begins, the baby is usually head down, lying slightly on one side with his spine pressed against the mother's abdominal wall. His head is flexed, chin pressed against his chest — this is the easiest way to accomplish the first part of the journey. As his body moves down, he twists and manoeuvres slightly, so that always his widest parts pass through the widest angles of the pelvis. With his head fully flexed, it passes easily

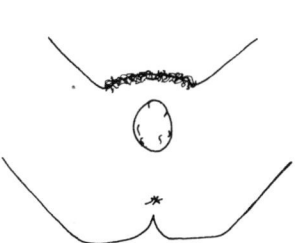

Fig.1 Perineum stretching

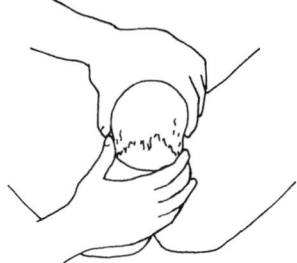

Fig.2 Head emerging

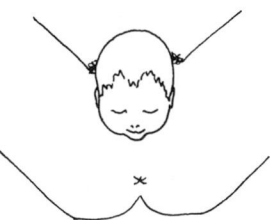

Fig.3 Head born and still extended

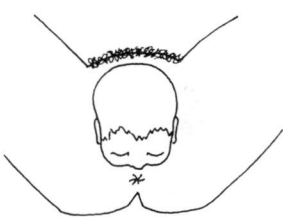

Fig.4 Head flexed

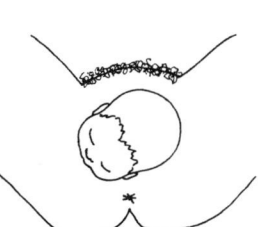

Fig.5 Restitution of head

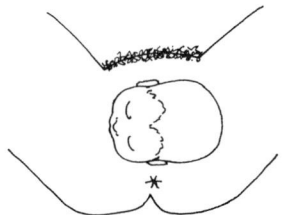

Fig.6 Rotation of head

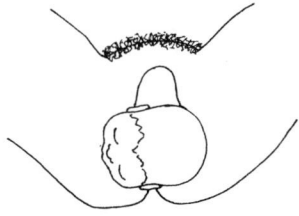

Fig.7 Birth of anterior [upper] shoulder

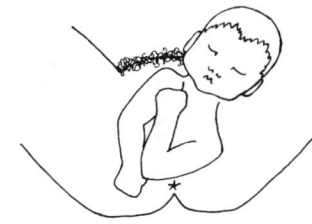

Fig.8 Birth of lower shoulder and body

under the mother's pubic bone soon after she begins to push. Then his head extends; he lifts his chin and arches his neck so that the top of his head is now going to press against the perineum, gradually stretching it and opening it up for delivery. When his head is born, his body will then turn either to the right or left (depending on which side he is lying) so that his shoulders will be born through the widest diameter of the pelvis. The rest of his body will slip easily through; the head and shoulders are his largest, least flexible parts.

RECOGNISING THE ONSET OF LABOUR

With first pregnancies, the baby's head becomes engaged in the pelvis up to four weeks before labour begins. The mother will become aware that there is less pressure under her ribs, breathing is easier at night, and pressure in the groin, especially against her bladder, is more noticeable. In subsequent pregnancies, the baby might not engage until labour commences.

The mucous plug is a gelatinous mass which plugs the cervix throughout pregnancy and protects the baby from vaginal bacteria. It comes away as the 'show' — small quantities of white or greyish mucous with traces of blood from the cervix. It may be eliminated several days before labour begins, or during the course of labour. So it is not necessarily a sign of imminent labour.

The membranes rupture spontaneously before labour begins in about 10% of pregnancies. Labour usually begins within hours if the baby is full term. The quantity of fluid lost varies from a few drops to three or four cupfuls, depending on the degree of engagement of the baby's head. If the head is well engaged, only the fluid trapped in front of the head will escape, with subsequent mild leaking. Amniotic fluid is produced continually by the body, so the baby continues to be cushioned in it even after the rupture; there is no such thing as the mythical "dry" delivery.

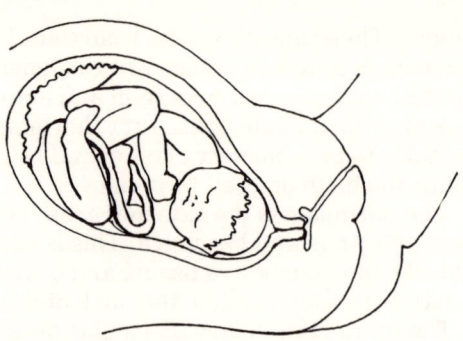

Fig.1 Full Term uterus — cervix not yet effaced or dilating.

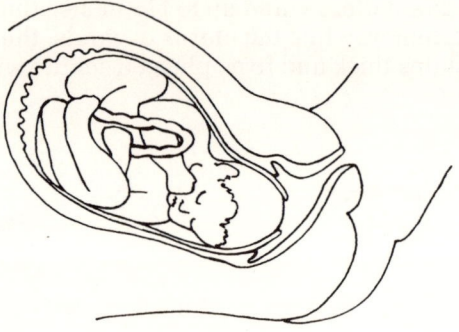

Fig.2 Cervix partly dilated — approx. 4 - 5 cms.

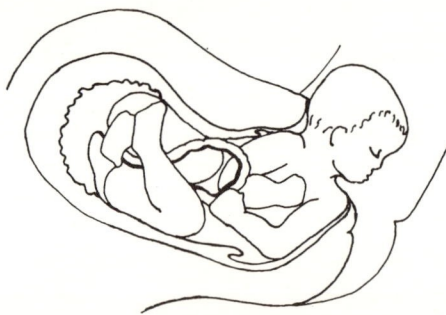

Fig.3 Cervix full dilated. Into Second Stage of Labour.

As labour approaches, women tend to find it easy to get things in order and see to last minute preparations, so they can relax and clear their heads of insignificant details — the modern day nesting instinct. In the final 24 hours, many women become aware of subtle differences; natural diarrhoea occurs as the body cleanses itself in preparation for labout; fairly heavy sensations similar to menstrual discomfort may be felt; and most noticeable will be the spurt of vigour as the body becomes energised for labour. Vaginal secretions increase significantly at the end of pregnancy. An internal examination at this point would usually show the cervix to be very soft, and possibly in the process of thinning out.

All signs of labour are exciting, but contractions are what gets the baby born, and are, therefore, the only really reliable indication that you are in labour. A contraction is generally felt as a tight, pulling sensation in the lower abdomen. When they occur regularly, becoming progressively stronger and closer together, labour can be considered established.

Sometimes labour seems to begin and then stops — discouragingly referred to as "false labour". When you are going to give birth at home there is no urgency to identify real labour, no fear of the inconvenience and disappointment of going into hospital just to be sent home again. Early labour that is slow to progress, or stops for a while, doesn't matter; flowing with it and not wishing anything otherwise comes naturally. Many women do experience one or two breaks in early labour. It is quite normal for the uterus to have warm-up, toning contractions before progressing into regular, progressively stronger, closer together contractions characteristic of established labour. In this early period, contractions may stop if you make a change from activity to rest or vice versa. You might be able to sleep through them in comfort, but when you are definitely in labour you will not be able to sleep through contractions, and they will persist no matter what you are doing.

The Birth of Nathan

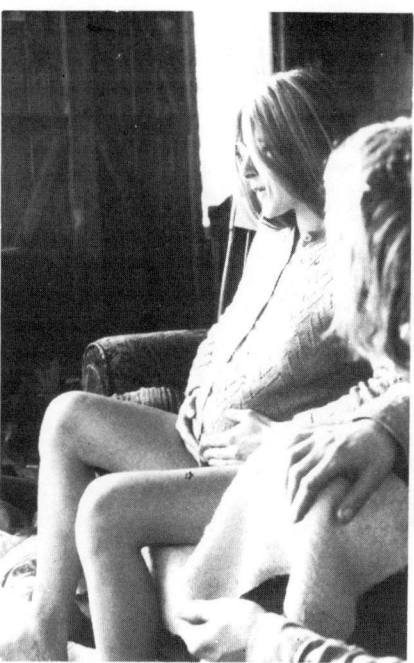

1 . . . . .

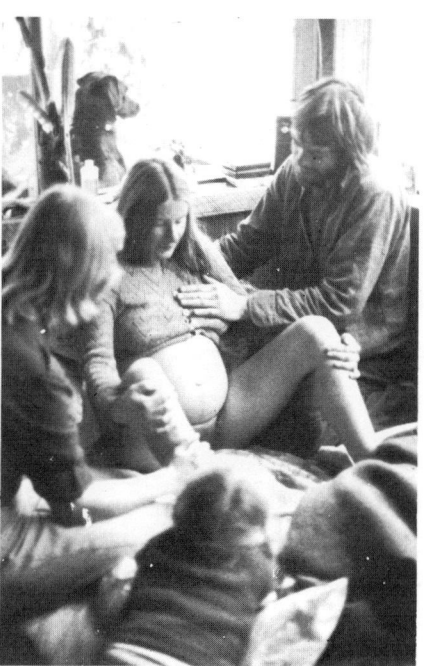

2 . . . . .

When contractions begin, you will probably feel overwhelmed in some way — excitement, the inevitability of the whole drama, and it is all going to happen right now! You may as well anticipate that labour will soon become established and prepare for it: have a meal that will supply energy reserves for both yourself and the baby, including food sources of potassium and vitamin K. Suitable foods are eggs, homemade bread, yoghurt, cheese, green vegetables and fruit. Also take 600 IU vitamin E, 1000mg vitamin C and extra calcium (preferably dolomite, as it is balanced with magnesium).

This combination raises the pain theshold, and the vitamin E gives added protection against brain-damage, should the baby be briefly deprived of oxygen during labor or delivery.

STAGES OF LABOUR

First Stage   The cervix effaces and dilates until the opening measures 10cm across. Labour contractions will be recognised as feeling different from Braxton-Hicks contractions. The dilation process is gradual; the body usually has plenty of time to adjust to its demands, making it easy to slip into control and maintain it when you need to. (A possible exception is a labour that follows a spontaneous rupture of the membranes; this is a natural induction and contractions may begin closer together and with speedier rise in intensity than usual. It is harder to adjust to this and more initial effort goes into control.) During this stage, the muscles at the top of the uterus push down on the baby's bottom, pressing the baby's head against the cervix. At the same time, the muscles in the lower segment of the uterus pull upwards; as the cervix is drawn open, the head pushes through, much as our own head pushes through a turtle-neck sweater.

Transition   This is still first stage labour,

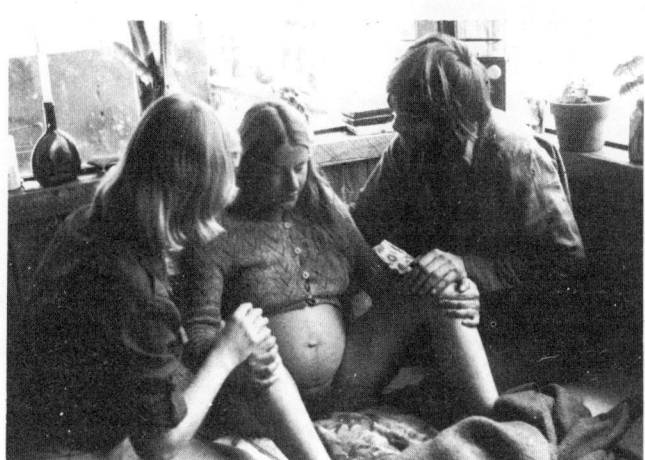

3 . . . . .

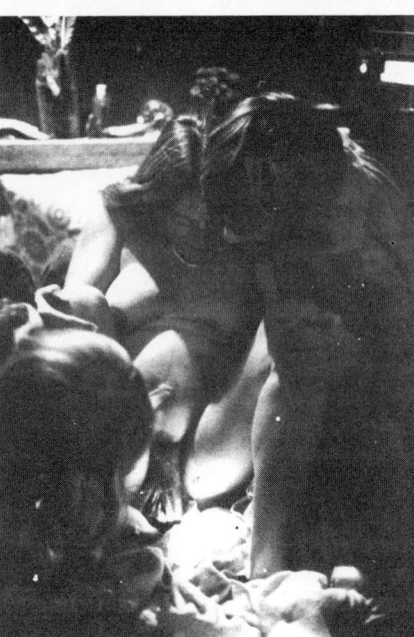

4 . . . . .

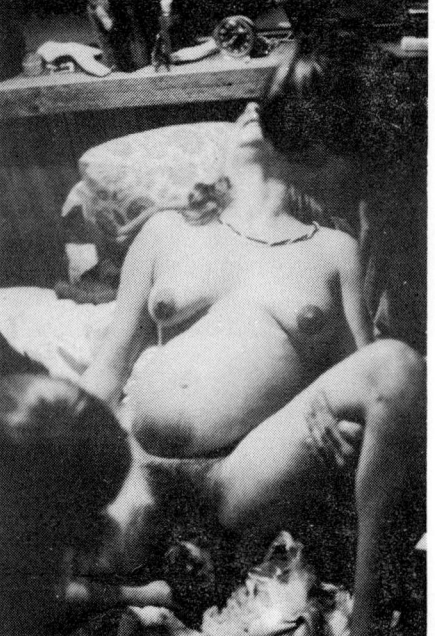

5 . . . . .

42

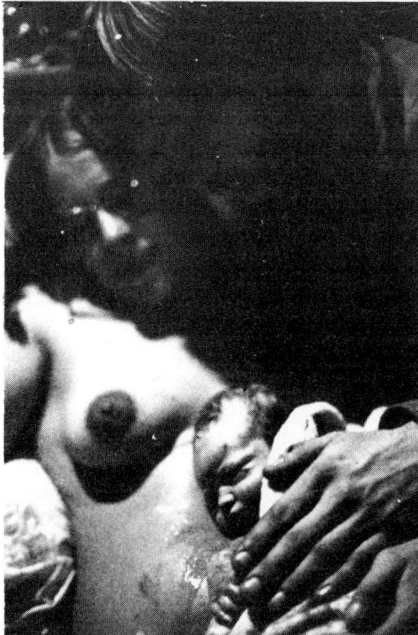

6 . . . . .

but a distinct change does occur at the end of the first stage, worth some attention.

The dilation from 7 or 8cm to the full 10cm tends to happen very quickly — from 5 to 45 minutes. These are the strongest contractions and they become irregularly spaced, some coming very close together.

The woman usually experiences a change in mood, resulting from sudden changes in hormonal levels and new hormones coming into play in preparation for the second stage. The body is thrown into a state of biological confusion, as intense efforts to complete one stage conflict with initial sensations of the next. Trembling or numbness, sudden feelings of cold, extreme or sudden tiredness, feelings of insecurity and inability to cope, irritability — all are sensations commonly experienced.

At this point, the baby's head is passed almost through the cervix and presses heavily on the tail-bone. This may feel like a huge need to move the bowels, and triggers a premature urge to push. Until the cervix is completely dilated, the urge to push must be suppressed as it would be painful, and there is a risk of tearing it. Controlling this urge, coupled with strong contractions and possible feelings of dejection and tiredness, is very difficult.

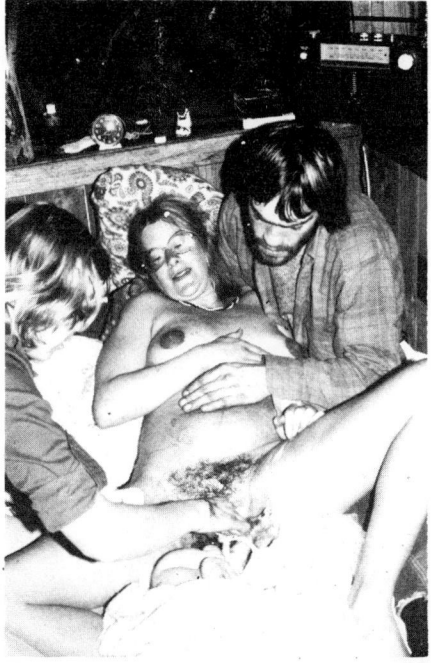

7 . . . . .

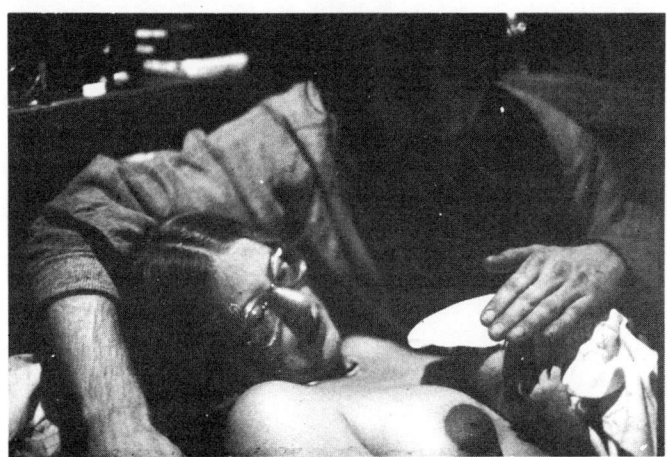

8 . . . . .

This stage should be anticipated and understood by all people involved with the birth.

While the sensations are unpleasant, there is a very positive side to it — it will be brief, and it heralds imminent birth. It is very much the time for taking one contraction at a time, as each one may be the last before everything changes. The father can give positive support throughout; maintaining eye contact with the woman will always keep her centered. He can be very positive and encouraging, in complete honesty, and the woman must learn beforehand that when he tells her she's in transition, she can accept his word and know that the baby is almost ready to be born.

A common question is: "When do you know when to push?" (without resorting to a vaginal examination). A short time — just a few minutes — after the cervix is fully dilated, the contractions become different; they are entirely expulsive and the difference may be apparent to the mother. The desire to push varies in intensity from person to person, but may well be uncontrollable at first — the body will begin to push regardless of whether or not the mother pushes. At this point, the mother will experience sudden and complete

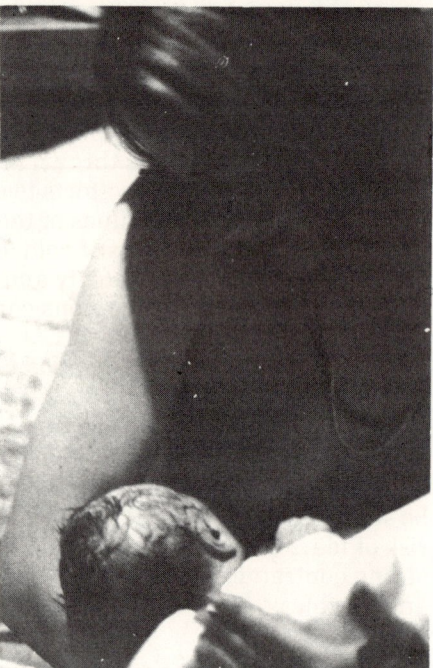

9 . . . . .

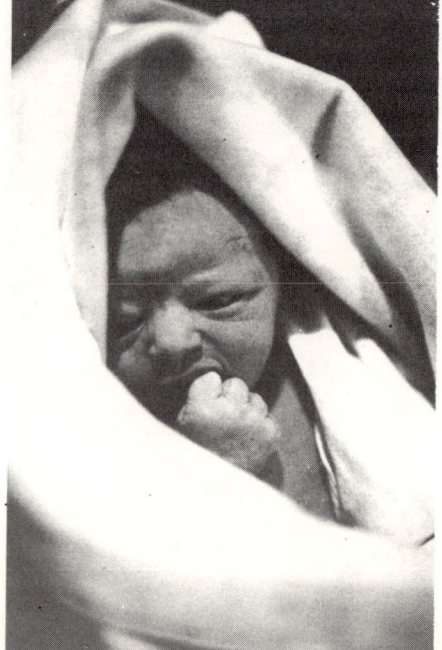

10

relief from her transition mood. A surge of energy will displace the tiredness. The atmosphere will change to eagerness and the whole room will 'catch' this energy. If you can control a couple of contractions while you are uncertain about transition being over, things will clarify in this time. If the woman squats at this time to make use of gravity, the baby will slip into the birth canal quite noticeably.

Second Stage   This is the expulsive phase, the baby's trip through the birth canal, and his birth. Contractions become more evenly spaced again with rest periods in between of several minutes. The pushing urge varies; it is overwhelmingly strong in some women, mild in others. Correct pushing is important and when properly done is very satisfying. This stage is quite painless for many women, except for a stretching, burning sensation in the perineum when the baby's head is nearly through.

As the baby's head passes through the cervix, the head is usually fully flexed (the chin is pressed against the chest). Like this, the head passes under the pubic bone, then it arches back so that the very top of the head is aiming at the vaginal outlet. At the same time, the baby's body turns so that the width of the shoulders will pass through the widest diameter of the bony pelvic outlet. Now contractions expel the baby's body from the uterus, each one pushing his head against the perineum. This persistent pressure dilates the opening and more and more of the head becomes visible. Soon the head will be through almost to the baby's ears, and the mother's skin can be eased back gently to let the head be born.

The midwife will support the baby's head, which will soon turn towards one of the mother's thighs. Now you will know which side the baby is facing and which shoulder will be born first — always the one on the same side as the baby's upper ear, and called the anterior shoulder. It is important to guide the upper shoulder out first and very gently, as tears in the perineum are more likely to occur with the birth of the shoulder than with the head. After the shoulders are out, the rest of the body may slip out easily, or the mother may need to push a little to help it. There is better control over the perineum if she does not push during the birth of the head and shoulders; the contractions alone exert ample pressure to do the job.

Delivery   These brief moments conclude the second stage of labour. The mother's work is almost done. The midwife supports the baby's head while the rest of the body is being born. While waiting for the next contraction, the baby's eyes may be wiped — separately — with sterile gauze pads. If time permits, the nostrils may be suctioned gently, especially if meconium has been passed in the fluid. Otherwise, beyond an instinctive move to lightly dry the face, you may wish to just wait. With the next contraction, guide the upper shoulder *slightly* downwards as it passes through (to get it under the mother's pubic bone) and then guide the baby upwards — *slightly* — to lead the lower shoulder out without pulling down unnecessarily on the mother's perineum. As the body follows, catch it into your arms taking care not to lessen the support of the head or jerk the spine in any way. Baby is used to being curled up and is easiest to hold with the spine again curved. It is a nice natural flow to guide the baby in an upward arc towards the belly of the mother, now soft and hollow — the perfect nest for the wee one. Do this slowly, just in case the cord is short or knotted.

Third Stage This is the birth of the pacenta (afterbirth) which occurs generally within 20 minutes after the baby. This is covered in detail later in this chapter.

MANAGEMENT OF LABOUR

How you spend your time during labour depends on yourselves, but there are a few points to remember in order to ensure a safe, easier labour.

1. The mother must pee every hour until she begins to deliver. A full bladder may not be noticed, there are many other dominating sensations, but a full bladder will interfere with the action of the uterus making contractions less effective and unnecessarily painful. A full bladder at the beginning of second stage is dangerous; it may prevent the baby from passing into the birth canal. Look at a diagram and see just where the bladder is, then you'll understand the importance of keeping it empty. A full bladder gets greatly traumatised during labour, and beyond interfering with labour, there may be many problems following labour. It is easy to pee every hour with all that pressure on the bladder, but women in labour lose track of time and it must be someone else's responsibility to remind her. Do it on the hour, or half hour, for easy remembering.

2. Listen to the baby's heartbeat every half hour once labour is established. You might find it easier to listen with your ear pressed to the abdomen. Stethoscopes are great at picking up all sounds and confusing the inexperienced ear. A fetuscope is best, but not absolutely necessary. Before labour begins, practice finding and counting the heartbeat. Once labour is established, mark the spot where you find it loudest; this will make it easier to relocate in between contractions. As the baby moves down the birth canal, so will that mark on the abdomen.

3. Time contractions; the best guide to the progress of labour is the strength of each contraction. Place your hand on the abdomen and you will quickly learn to estimate the strength. You may detect a kind of pattern to them — a few strong ones followed by a more mild one at regular intervals. Take contractions one at a time; it is not reasonable to worry about the next ones if you have trouble controlling one, as the next one will not automatically be a stronger one still. If you can handle one, you can handle them all. The test is rather one of endurance and very important is being prepared for each one. Rest and relax in between, but DO NOT sleep, unless someone is with you constantly to wake you in time to get some good, deep, cleansing breaths before a contraction begins.

4. Once labour is well established, all body energy is directed to the uterus; circulation to the lower limbs is reduced to a minimum so warm sox will be appreciated. The digestive system slows right down, so don't eat heavy foods once labour is going well, or it will sit heavily in your stomach and possibly make you nauseated. Just snack lightly if you feel like it. Lemon drinks or teas sweetened with honey are refreshing, nice on your throat, and quite energising.

5. Watch the mother's condition. Usually a glance will tell you she is in fine shape and you won't have to take any evaluative measures. Some tiredness is to be expected, and this is likely to become pronounced during transition. Fears, doubts and anxieties are also normal reactions, but are problems to be worked out rather than being threatening situations.

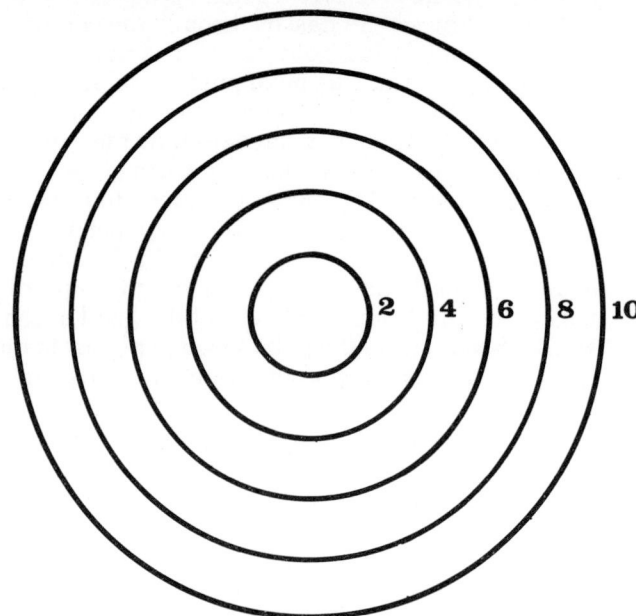

Dilation of Cervix in Centimeters.

6. Vaginal examinations should not be attempted by an inexperienced person. Besides the risk of introducing infection, it takes a lot of practice to get to know what you are feeling. Rectal examinations are safer from the point of view of infection, but it is even more difficult to know what you are feeling. Do not attempt either kind yourself, and if a midwife chooses to do them, the fewer done the better. If labour is progressing satisfactorily, there is no need to do them. In *Commonsense Childbirth*, Lester Hazell describes how to follow the progress of labour without internal examinations, and I strongly endorse this approach.

7. Begin boiling instruments when labour is going strong.

8. Have the birth area prepared during strong labour, as it will be needed any time after transition begins.

If you are birthing without professional help, try not to get caught up in the heaviness of the responsibility; the real heavy lies in your decision to birth at home and in your preparations for the event. By the time you get into labour, you must be completely comfortable with your decision, and confident in your preparations. Your trust in each other must be complete.

Women experience a different consciousness when they are really into labour. Everyone present should respect this. Do not violate the privacy of her mood, especially if she and her man are in close communion, clearly flowing with the labour. Hospitalised women tend to withdraw into themselves in an attempt to escape distractions; it is as if avoiding one distraction, they have to avoid them all, and the father feels excluded. Often he learns afterwards that his presence was highly valued and depended on, but his actual experience was one of uncertainty and mere hope that he was doing all the right things.

This exclusion should not happen at home, and should be discouraged if it does happen. It is the one valid occasion on which to break the mother's mood and, when done sensitively, will probably help her. The sense of sharing is an important one during labour and birth. The more fully she can share, the less likely she is to get into inhibiting state of aloneness, uncertainty, hostility or fear. Sharing it with her man ensures that the occasion remains joyful, magical, a time for laughter as much as seriousness. The atmosphere must allow her to be herself; she does not have to fit the tight-lipped, intensely controlled, "successful", Lamaze image; she must be free to express her emotions. She is a very real person doing a very real thing, and she most certainly WILL have emotions! In transition especially, her mate might have to work at keeping these emotions positive, and guide her in a way he senses is best for her. Some women require deep eye-to-eye contact and silent concentration; others like to holler — not through loss of control, but because this releases their tensions. A holler that ends with a grin or giggle is fine; flow with it. Hollers indicating fear or distress and which inhibit the progress of labour, will be clearly distinguishable and warrant some mood-changing therapy.

Perineal Support During Birth   In North America the episiotomy is a routine procedure. In most other civilised countries, it is done only when considered necessary — a small percentage, usually for breech deliveries and complicated ones requiring the use of forceps. Premature deliveries sometimes require a small episiotomy, as the tissues have not become fully elasticised. The number of normal, uncomplicated, full term deliveries requiring an episiotomy is very, very few. Even these might have had a different outcome if time was spent in encouraging and relaxing the mother. Perineal support is often not practiced by hasty doctors who prefer to slit it instead.

There is an art to good support, but it is easily learned when you understand what it does.

Delivery without episiotomy or tears is a result of several responsibilities being carried out. The mother assists her tissues to become fully elastic and controllable in both her vitamin C and E intake, and her muscle control exercises, and then, by effective control of her pushing during the second stage. The midwife contributes by conducting the birth in a calm, unhurried manner, working in unison with the mother during contractions and supporting the perineum as the baby's head bulges against it, to prevent the head from bursting through, uncontrolled. Similar guidance is needed for the birth of the shoulders.

As the head emerges through the birth canal, it pushes against the fleshy perineum and the vulva, bulging them out and thinning them. The labia separates and the crown of the head begins to appear in the opening. At first it will slip back out of sight in between contractions; but when quite a lot of head is showing, it will remain visible. It is at this point that it becomes important to support the perineum.

Place a sterile, square, gauze pad in the palm of your right hand (unless you are left-handed). Place this palm flat against the perineum, squarely between the anus and the vulva. Spread your thumb and forefinger to cup the now-bulging vulva and control the skin around the lower edge of the vagina. The gauze gives you traction, as skin on skin tends to get slippery. In between contractions throughout second stage labour, massage the perineum with vitamin E oil. The massage, the vitamin and the lubrication all help tremendously.

During contractions, let the baby's head push into your palm. The amount of counter-pressure you exert is important. You must allow the baby's head to progress a little with each contraction and continue to dilate the opening, but you also have to stop it bursting through before the skin is fully stretched. Too much pressure will be painful on the mother's distended anus, especially if she has haemorrhoids. The mother must co-operate by not bearing down, thus letting the head be born more slowly. You will feel instinctively when to let the head slip through — the whole crown will be showing and you'll probably not be able to hold it back without alarming pressure. At this point continue your right-handed support, and with the fingers of your left hand draped down over the head, guide it out with both hands in a slightly upward movement. The baby will be face down while the crowning takes place, and at the birth of the head, the neck will extend and the face will appear as the lower section of the vaginal outlet slides down to reveal brow, eyes, nose, mouth and chin. Very soon the head will rotate to one side and you can easily support it in one hand while feeling for the cord around the neck.

If a tear occurs, it will usually happen when the shoulders are born (birth of the shoulders is not difficult, but they are wide). Let them be born smoothly; slightly draw the baby downward to bring the upper shoulder out from under the pubic bond, then guide the baby upward and the lower shoulder and body will follow through.

Any tear will likely be down the middle of the perineum, along the natural join line. Up to half an inch long is of no surgical consequence; any more than that may require suturing. This is best done within 12 hours, but is not an immediate problem. Comfrey compresses from strong tea will promote swift healing. Natural tears are not particularly uncomfortable compared to a surgical cut. Doctors loathe repairing a ragged edge, but that ragged edge means less cell damage and easier healing. Also, a natural tear involves only skin and mucous membrane over a small area; American-style episiotomies average a two inch cut through membrane, muscle tissue, nerves, blood vessels and skin. Scar tissue following episiotomy repair inhibits the elasticity of the area for future births.

APGAR Assessment of the Newborn

Hospitals routinely use this method of evaluating the newborn's general condition, and you may feel more comfortable understanding this assessment. It is ironical that a hosptial baby is more likely to need this immediate evaluation as its birth is so often stresful and complicated. Yet within hospitals, this assessment

APGAR Assessment

60 Sec.   5 Mins.

A - appearance (colour)
- 2 if the skin is completely pink
- 1 if body is pink, and limbs or feet are bluish
- 0 if entire body is blue

P - pulse
- 2 if above 100 per minute
- 1 if less than 100 per minute
- 0 if pulse/heartbeat is absent

G - grimace* (annoyed response to suctioning or stroking the sole of the foot)
- 2 if cries vigorously
- 1 if grimaces or cries a little
- 0 if no response

A - activity*
- 2 if making active motions
- 1 if some leg/arm movement
- 0 if motionless and limp

R - respiration (breathing)
- 2 if strong efforts to breathe
- 1 if breathing slow and irregular
- 0 if not breathing

Baby's Name ....
Date ....

TOTALS: _____

*The baby may be quite relaxed after a calm birth; there will be no vigorous protests to calculate from, and no desire on your part to stimulate any. You can estimate these points by observing tentative, explorative movements the baby will make — even a relaxed baby makes involuntary unco-ordinated movements. If this is happening, you won't need to provoke the child, especially if the score for the other signs is good. In hospital, the baby is usually protesting a catheter stuck down his throat, a slap on the bottom, or being dangled by his ankles.

Apart from counting the pulse, the rest falls into your general appraisal of the child. Have an APGAR chart drawn up ahead of time and call out your scores to the person handling it. Here is a sample chart for easy use; just tick beside the appropriate description.

(See Pages 92-96 for additional APGAR Charts)

is becoming increasingly unreliable, as it is now known that certain drugs, particularly Demerol, depress a baby in several ways which are apparent within the first four days of life; yet the APGAR scores of these babies do not indicate their true condition. However, following unmedicated birth, the assessment will be very accurate.

The baby is assessed on five vital newborn signs. Each sign is given a score using a scale of 0 to 2. A score of 2 indicates the baby fully demonstrates that particular sign; 1 indicates a partial response; 0 means that particular sign is absent.

The assessment is carried out 60 seconds after the birth and again five minutes later. A total score of 7 to 10 is considered good; the baby will survive without help. A score of 4, 5, or 6 indicates some immediate assistance is needed to help him get started; suctioning and gentle touch stimulation is generally enough — a mucous blockage is often the problem. The baby with a score of less than 4 is the problem baby. This baby is limp, pale, unresponsive, possibly not breathing, and may even lack a heartbeat. Intensive assistance, artificial respiration, is necessary to get the baby working on his own.

Most babies score 7 to 10 at 60 seconds, and a full 10 at the five minute assessment. Nine or ten is common in undrugged, normal births at the 60 second assessment.

How to do an APGAR Assessment   Get a third person to watch the clock and time the moment of birth, then inform you of the one and five minute intervals after that moment. The same person can record your assessment.

If any questions about your homebirth are raised later on, the APGAR assessment may indicate some degree of responsibility, concern and preparation on your part. It may also be useful information for a doctor if the child later needs medical treatment.

The First ten Minutes   For a short while there is nothing to be done. Baby will wail once or twice with his first breaths, sometimes before his body is born, sometimes after. A healthy baby is blue at birth and has good muscle tone — he resists your touch and pushes against you. The colour changes to a purplish-red with his initial breaths, and then a pink wave will flush right through his body. You need adequate light (but not harsh light) to see this, and also to watch the movement of his spine as he breathes, both for the baby's safety and for your own peace of mind.

He will probably establish himself so quickly and easily you'll be left feeling totally unnecessary, with a head full of emergency procedures for which there is no need. For up to ten minutes, time will be filled with the wonder and realisation of birth, the excitement of a new daughter or son. It is a natural time for family closeness, emotionally, physically, and spiritually.

Within ten minutes the cord will probably be limp, no longer pulsing, no longer a necessary link for the baby. You can now cut it at your leisure. Tie the cord tightly in two places, an inch apart, the tie nearest to the baby being two inches from his abdomen. Cut in between the ties. Most babies like to explore the breast at this time, although not all begin to nurse actively right away.

Delivery of the Placenta   After the cord is cut, you may feel some milder contractions. If you squat over a basin and push gently, the placenta will probably be born. It is a small, flexible mass and its birth will cause no discomfort.

The placenta may present in one of two ways. Most commonly the shiny fetal surface is turned outermost and the membranes trail behind it (like am umbrella blown inside out). It is easy to catch the placenta in both hands and gently twist it as the membranes trail out so they come out intact. In about 25% of births, the placenta does not turn inside out, but slides out with the raw surface which was attached to the uterine wall outermost. There is a greater chance of a part being left behind when this happens, so it must be delivered slowly and carefully, then closely examined for completeness.

"Midwifery" by Jean Hallum, on pages 56 and 57 describes and illustrates these two methods of separation, while pages 32 and 33 describe and illustrate the parts and variations in placentas.

The placenta is a fantastic structure; it invites wonder and fascination. Disposing of it is like parting with a friend. Eating it is a very good thing to do — if you can — as it rapidly makes up for any blood loss during the birth. Count the blood vessels in the cord; there should be *three*. This is important. In rare cases there are only two, and internal abnormalities in the child are usually associated with this.

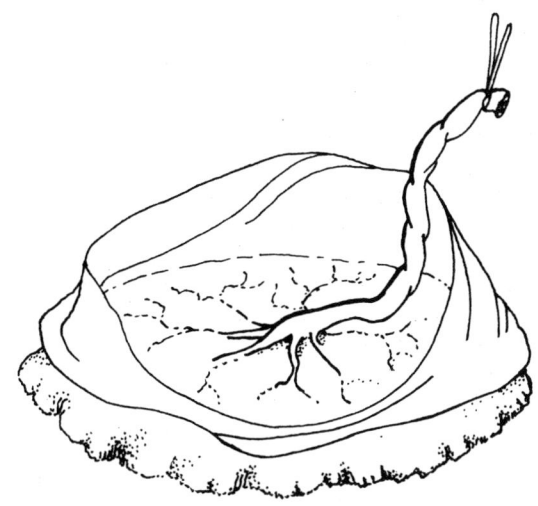

Fig.1

— Reading —

Hazell, Lester.   Commonsense Childbirth

Hallum, Jean.   Midwifery

Lang, Raven.   Birth Book

Also refer to diagrams listed at the end of the Appendix called 'Problem Solving'.

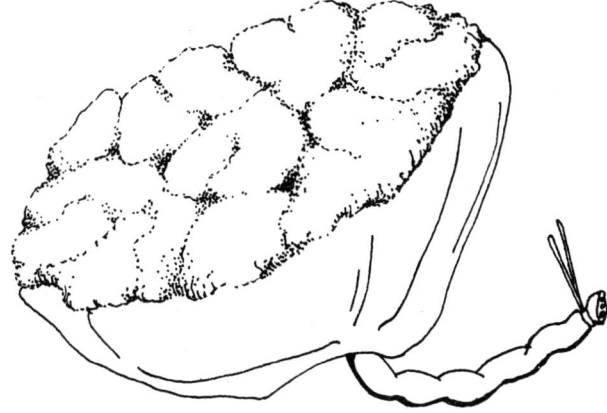

The Placenta

Fig.1 Fetal surface and bag of membranes.

Fig.2 Maternal surface.

Fig.2

Labour and Delivery Sheet

Stage		Symptoms	Duration	Mother	Father or Midwife	Friend	Supplies
Approaching Labour		Slight weight loss. Baby may engage. Increased pressure. Vaginal discharge; energy spurt.	Last 2 - 3 weeks Last 24 - 36 hours				
Onset of Labour		'Show' and/or waters rupture and/or contractions.	Individual signs may occur within 2 weeks of due date.	Conserve energy. Warn birth attendants.	Cut fingernails? Share a light meal.		
First Stage	Early	Regular contractions, 10 - 25 minutes apart, 45 - 60 seconds long.	2 - 7 hours [variable]	Walk; light housework. First level breathing when needed.	Begin timing contractions. Listen to baby half-hourly. Make mother pee every hour.	Get supplies ready. Start boiling the things and prepare the birth area. Have fluids available for mother, and cool face-cloths.	Pencil and Paper.
First Stage	Advanced	Contractions 5 minutes apart, 60 seconds long.	½ - 2 hours [variable]	Second level breathing and effleurage. Conscious relaxation.	As above. More moral support needed during contractions. Check mother's relaxation.		
First Stage	Transition	Contractions 1 - 2 minutes apart, 60 - 90 seconds long. May feel shaky, anxious, tired, hot or cold, irritable, nausea. Urge to push.	Between 5 - 15 contractions [up to ¾ hour].	Try kneeling or squatting. Stay awake and aware in spite of tiredness.	Constant support and encouragement; eye-to-eye contact. Make sure mother recognises where she is at. Be ready to get scrubbed-up for delivery soon.		Delivery set must be sterilised and handy. Sterile sheet on bed. Zephiran or other antiseptic.
Second Stage		Urge to push may intensify. Rest of transition symptoms disappear. New energy burst. Contractions allow 2 - 3 good pushes each; longer rest periods.	10 - 60 minutes. If longer, check pushing technique and try a new position.•	Squat; or sit slightly reclined against back support. Push with contractions until head crowns. Blow through 2 - 3 delivery contractions. Keep face and bottom relaxed!	Support perineum during contractions, massaging in between. After the head crowns, ease it through gently pushing perineum back. Feel and look for cord. [If around neck, loosen it, or clamp it in two places and cut it]. Continue to support the head. Ease upper shoulder out with contraction, catch baby into your arms.	Be with mother while husband goes to scrub-up for delivery. Support her body. Note time of birth. Prepare to record first APGAR Test.	Have clamps and scissors handy.

Third Stage	Duration	Symptoms	Do APGAR assessment at 60 seconds and at 5 minutes after the birth.		Baby
	15 mins to 2 hours	Mild contractions; gush of blood as placenta separates.	Nurse the baby. Squat and push to expel the placenta.	Catch the placenta; ease it out slowly and twist the trailing membranes. Assess the blood loss and check uterus for hardness.	Allow baby to uncurl on mother's belly; let him play at her breast. Keep him close to your body for warmth - use soft wraps. If you don't do APGAR scores, watch his general responses, his breathing and colour. Baby should be pink, aware and making some tentative, exploratory movements within minutes of birth.

		Observations of:		
		Mother	Child	Other
Post-Partum	First 2 hours after birth	Keep a close check on blood loss. Clean up after the placenta is born — loss then should look like a heavy period. Feel uterus often [at least every 15 minutes] Massage it if not hard like a grapefruit.	Check cord stump frequently; retie it if the original tie becomes slack. Check that baby continues to breathe easily; unhindered by mucous. Baby should be pink all over; ears, fingertips, lips, etc. Will be nursing strongly within the first hour.	Examine placenta for completeness; also the membranes. Count the number of blood vessels in the cord — there should be three. The Le Boyer bath?
Post-Partum	First few days	The mother does not need to be bedridden at all, but does need to take it easy. Recovery can be too quick for her own good, so that on the third or fourth days she is strung out from being too busy. Lochia [discharge] will fade to pink in 2 - 3 days, then become watery; it will clear up in about two weeks, more or less. If it gets foul smelling, or you get feverish, get help to ward off possible infection. The baby needs sensible care; no chills or drafts. Take him for a medical exam within the first couple of weeks, or sooner if you are worried. He should pee and pass meconium within 24 hours. Remember to register him, get a birth certificate, and claim the child allowance!		

Mothercare

The midwife will stay at least two hours after the birth; if you are without a midwife, the mother's body must not be forgotten in the excitement. Any haemorraging is most likely to occur in the first two hours. Once the placenta is born, the uterus contracts strongly and does an amazing shrink to about grapefruit size and hardness within minutes. You can feel it by prodding the stomach just above the pubic bone (this prodding does not hurt or cause any damage). The mother should quickly learn to recognise how it should feel so she can check it herself every 15 minutes for the first two or three hours, then frequently over the next day or two. If it softens, gentle massage or the baby nursing will usually firm it up right away. If the mother feels fine, a shower can be taken; someone must stay constantly with her as she may be weak from the sudden changes in her body, blood loss and having used up an unusual amount of energy. She may prefer someone to give her a refreshing sponge bath. Giver her two sanitary napkins to wear, as the blood loss is like a heavy period to begin with.

For the first few days, the bleeding (lochia) remains like a heavy period, but after a week, the discharge will be considerably less and more pinkish and watery. This in turn will go clear brownish as it tapers off. At no point should the discharge look murky or smell offensive. This is a sign of infection and will probably be accompanied by fever and general discomfort, and requires antibiotic treatment immediately. Until your body is fully recovered, you must be really fussy about personal hygiene. Shower or sponge-bath while the discharge persists; after using the toilet, wipe from front to back to avoid rectal contamination.

Commence pelvic-floor muscle contractions right away after the birth and continue to do them a lot. Initially you may not feel anything happening as the area us numbed from the birth, nonetheless, they are most important to get your pelvic-floor back into good shape.

Mothers recuperating at home are very different from our social image of a newly delivered woman. Being undrugged and not having an episiotomy makes a huge difference. Particularly if it is not her first birth, and the labour was comparatively fast and 'easy', the mother may not act like she has just given birth — except for her obvious emotional high. I

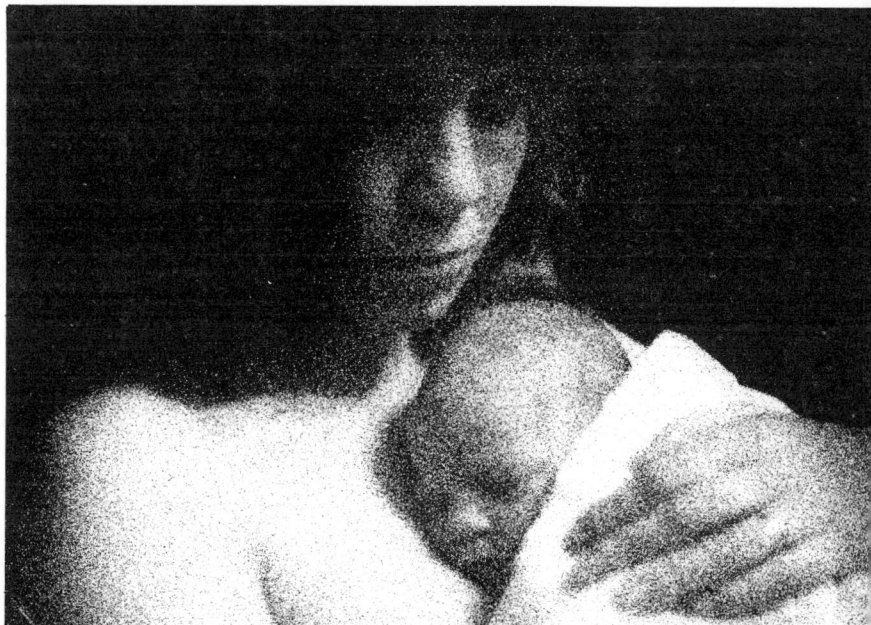

Ingrid and baby Galen

recall, after an exceptionally brief second stage with our son, being left with an enormous amount of unused energy. If the mother can possibly rest she should do so. A wonderful advantage to being at home is that resting is not confined to bed; it can be done in an easy chair before a log fire, or on a deck-chair in the sun. Fresh air and sunlight are the perfect complement to these emotional highs, the perfect energy source for soothing and healing. If you have the privacy to do so, expose your body to the sun. It is marvellous for nipples trying to adjust to the sudden onslaught of sucking, and your bottom will appreciate some fresh air and freedom from pads. It is good for your tummy if you can lie on it for a while each day; put a pillow under it and wherever else you need to keep your weight off your breasts.

On about the third day, sensation makes a comeback and your bottom may feel a little more tender than previously. There is usually some degree of bruising and tissue trauma during birth even if you didn't tear.

Involution of the Uterus

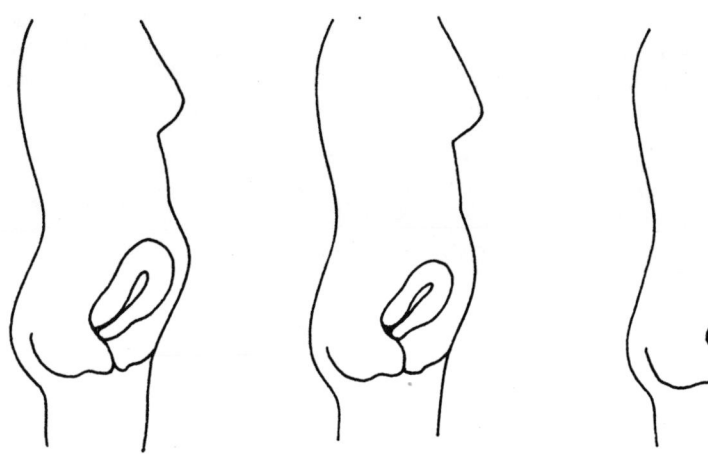

Fig.1 After the birth   Fig.2 One Week after the Birth.   Fig.3 Six weeks after the Birth — uterus returned to non-pregnant size.

If you suffered haemorrhoids during delivery, they may become uncomfortable now. Pads soaked in warm ginger tea or comfrey tea are healing and soothing. Crushed cranberry (even frozen cranberries will do) poultices relieve the pain of haemorrhoids. If you have had haemorrhoids, you should be taking Rutin, 30mg three times a day, to cure them — this really works well. (Rutin is a bioflavanoid, a substance found in nature in close conjunction with vitamin C). Drink comfrey tea to aid general internal healing; Golden Seal is another very healing herb, though it is nauseating in all but small amounts.

During the first few days you may be aware of your uterus as it continues to contract. "After-pains" are more bothersome in subsequent pregnancies, and are mostly felt when the baby nurses. Continued supplements of Calcium and vitamin E should make it easier. At first you will be aware, too, of fresh bleeding each time the baby nurses, caused by these contractions.

Most Important: Do not be tempted to take aspirin, or any preparation containing Salicylate. For one thing, by the time the drug becomes effective, the cramps are usually gone. More importantly, the drug passes to the baby through the breast milk. Aspirin may cause internal bleeding in babies of any age. The newborn does not manufacture his own vitamin K (the substance which allows his blood to clog) until his eighth day, and thus is much more susceptible to bleeding at this time. Also, Salicylates combine with albumin, which the baby needs to combine with bilirubin during the breakdown of the excess fetal blood cells. So aspirin taken at this time may cause jaundice, or make it worse.

The first few weeks following a birth are special family time, whether it is the first baby or the fifth. Do not do unnecessary work, use the time to rest or simply *be* with the family. The mother, in spite of feeling really well, must remember that her body is still busy. Her

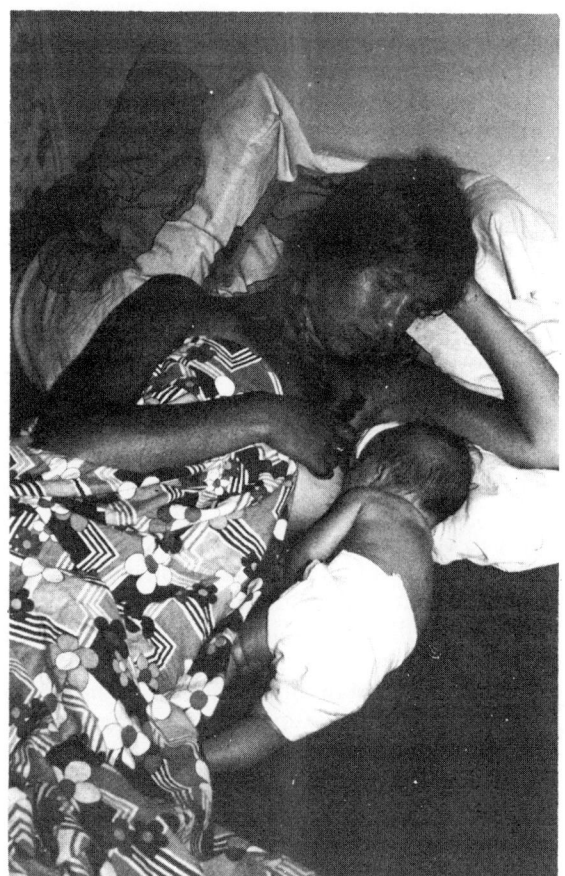

reproductive organs are still returning to normal non-pregnany status. Her body is using a lot of energy as it nourishes her child, catering to an ever-increasing demand for milk(this tends to be overlooked if the breastfeeding experience is smooth and comfortable). If you do overdo things, it will catch up with you; you'll feel suddenly tired, even exhausted, and have a fussy baby, too, if your milk supply is affected — all when your husband has gone back to work. So it is well worth the luxury of accepting any help offered in the first few weeks regardless of how great you feel.

The Newborn

The child, still naked, should be held against her mother's body; she will probably be toying with the breast and gazing intently at her parents' faces. Her ability to focus immediately after birth is powerful. Cover her back and head with a warm towel to prevent heat loss; room temperature should be 72-75°F (22-24°C). Following an uncomplicated birth, the baby will be an all-over, healthy, pink-red colour and breathing fairly regularly. Once the afterbirth is born and the mother is made comfortable, time belongs to the new family alone.

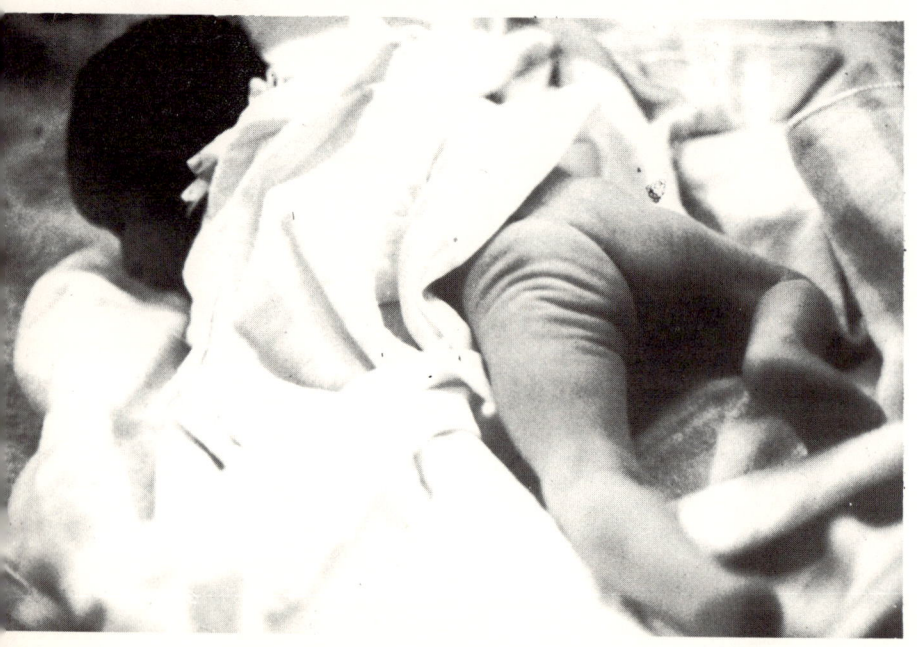

Birth itself is an experience many parents choose to share, and is a joyful time of outgoing energy. But don't be surprised if, quite soon after the birth, you begin to feel a need to be alone and undistracted by the company of friends. As the bonding experience takes place, the parents must be free to be alone with the child; this time is extremely precious and special; others might even sense the need to retreat, and can perhaps prepare food and tea in the kitchen for a while, staying within earshot in case they are needed.

The parents may choose to immerse the child in warm water (LeBoyer could improve his technique only by insisting that the parents do this — the communion that takes place is truly sacramental, and does *not* belong to the doctor!) The water must be blood-temperature, 98°F. It is simply to provide a familiar, weightless experience, simulating the security of the womb, and babes quite visibly relax and enjoy it, usually bestowing their first smiles as they lie back in a perfect physical and spiritual environment. Parents experience bonding as perhaps the most profound, enlightening moment of their lives. The babe who has undergone the stress (not distress) of labour and birth without being hurt or frightened, now begins to feel strong physical pleasure as her instincts begin to be felt — the sucking urge, the eye-to-eye contact — and as all her needs are met; she experiences deep love and security; she desires to keep on letting in new experiences and sensations, and is happy to greet her life head-on.

The newborn is an exquisite little thing, with all senses functioning and dynamic powers of communication. The home setting greatly enhances your ability to feel and perceive her fully; the calm birth and heartfelt welcome allows the baby to show her true self. She will be an alert, bright-eyed little person, very sensitive to sound.

The bonding process involves more than the sense of sight. Sound and touch and smell are also important means for indentification. The newborn responds instantly to the smell of a mother's skin, as much by the way she holds her and the kind of loving sounds they invoke in each other. It is kindest to the little one, therefore, to minimise unnecessary and confusing smells, like soap, disinfectant, incense and smoke for as long as possible. She will be very sensitive to the atmosphere of her birth place, and responsive to all she comes into contact with. Both our children were awake and curious, seemingly intent on examining our faces and immediate surroundings, for 2 to 3 hours after birth, before slowly drifting into a calm, deep sleep.

The law in some countries [*not New Zealand*] requires that all babies born in a hospital be treated to safeguard against gonoccocal eye infection, which causes blindness if not treated. Silver nitrate drops are the usual treatment. This law does not apply to babies born outside of hospitals, and so, if you are sure there is no medical risk, you don't need to do anything. If either parent has ever had, or could have had gonococcal infection, you must get a suitable antibiotic eye ointment to treat the baby's eyes. Do not use silver nitrate; the active ingredient is nitric acid. It burns the baby's eyes and kills off all bacteria, good and bad, so that until the necessary, healthy bacteria manage to grow back, the baby has no resistance to eye infections. The eyes become red and puffy, and the baby becomes the living myth; puffy-eyed, screwed-up face, unable to focus, and unhappy. Antibiotic treatment is painless and effective. The difference is that it must be used at regular intervals over a period of time. Silver nitrate is instilled only once; therefore it is easier on hospital staff to dump the acid and then forget about it.

Expressed breast milk is also good for cleansing and curing mucky eyes.

SUBSEQUENT CARE

In the hours following the birth, check periodically that the baby remains pink all over; hands, feet, lips, ears, all should be pink. Check that the cord stump is not bleeding. You may need to tie it with a new piece of sterile gauze if the stump has shrunk, making the original tie loose. Dab alcohol around the base of the cord (a cotton bud does the job best) and continue to do this at every diaper change until the cord drops off — usually in six to ten days.

Never expose the baby to chill or drafts; this is one thing she cannot handle. Keep the room temperature at a constant, sensible level which is comfortable for you (around 70-72°F). The newborn's liver is still immature and does not regulate the baby's temperature right away. She will be at room temperature, regardless of the amount of clothing or number of blankets you use. Within two or three weeks the baby will radiate her own warmth, and you'll be quite aware of it when it happens.

Any fever is abnormal, as is any discharge from the cord. Try to keep the cord stump from getting too urine-soaked. Baby powders are not a good idea as they can irritate sensitive skin and have been known to contain tetanus spores. Cornstarch is a cheap, more effective substitute to use on her bottom.

The newborn will nurse every few hours around the clock. The Colostrum, or first milk, she receives at this time is rich in vitamins and other essential nutrients, and is especially important in providing resistance to diseases, which is a life-long benefit. She will nurse frequently, partly to get this essential nourishment, partly because she has a strong instinct to suck and establish her milk supply, and partly because to do so is a great source of security, comfort and pleasure. The close physical and spiritual contact of the nursing couple extends and deepens the bonding between them.

There is seldom anything wrong with the child who continues to remain a good colour, sucks well, and breathes normally. It will be obvious right away whether or not the child is physically perfect. If you don't have a doctor or midwife at the birth to do a competent examination of the child, it would be wise to arrange a medical check-up sometime in the first couple of weeks. The doctor will listen in to the chest, the heart and lungs, and will check the other internal organs by palpation. He will examine ears and eyes, gums and palate, the genitals, her normal reflexes, her hips and spine.

You can do a certain amount of checking for yourself initially. Average newborn statistics and vital signs are as follows:

Weight   From 6lbs and up to 9 or 10lbs; the majority of babies nowadays from good nutritional backgrounds average 7 to 9 lbs. A baby 5 - 5½lbs or less is considered small for term, or premature, and should be handled with extra consideration and great care to see that she is kept warm and thrives normally. Unless the child develops a breathing problem, the small or slightly premature child will thrive best at home on breastmilk and lots of love and gentle cuddling.

Length   At term, the average length is 19-21 inches, although large variations are common.

Temperature   Rectally, it should be 98-99.5°F (36.5 - 37.5°C).

Pulse   Generally it is between 130 and 160 per minute, but this can vary even more depending on how relaxed, or active, she is at the time. You can best feel the pulse at the baby's wrist or in her groin, or else use the stethoscope if you have one.

Breathing   The baby breathes rapidly, about 60 to 70 times a minute for the first couple of hours after the birth, then it settles down to between 40 and 60 breaths a minute. It is several weeks before her breathing becomes completely regular, so if you are watching or listening to her as she sleeps, don't be alarmed if irregular periods occur, or the occasional breath is missed altogether. Unless the breathing looks or sounds difficult and laboured, there is no problem.

Weight Gain   A weight loss of 4 to 6 ounces usually occurs in the first two or three days as the amount the baby ingests is less than the amount passed through her kidneys and bowels. As the milk supply comes in, weight is gained and she may regain her birth weight by the end of the first week.

Jaundice   About two-thirds of newborns develop jaundice to some degree on the second or third day, and it may last just a day or two, a week at the most. Babies are born with an excess of red blood cells which begin to break down after the birth, and the end product of this process is called Bilirubin, which the body then eliminates. If this cell breakdown occurs very rapidly, the bilirubin will not be eliminated at the same rate, and will accumulate in the baby's tissues, giving it a jaundiced — yellow — appearance. You should have safeguarded against this by taking vitamin E supplements during pregnancy and labour, and the baby continues to get it through both colostrum and the breastmilk. With this precaution, any jaundice will likely be mild, lasting only a day or so. Severe jaundice can do irreversible brain damage; if you can see yellow in the baby's palms or the soles of her feet and she appears lethargic, then you should get advice and a blood bilirubin level test done. Exposure to sunlight (with care to protect her eyes and prevent her from burning) will help reduce the jaundice; just expose her for five minutes at a time, outdoors or through closed windows. (See chapter, Mother care, for special note regarding the use of Aspirin.)

Abnormal Jaundice Jaundice which occurs at, or soon after birth — within 24 hours, or appearing after the fifth day, cannot be normal, physiological jaundice; get medical attention

Vaginal Bleeding A small spotting of bright blood may be passed by a female child on the third or fourth day. This is normal, caused by maternal hormones transferred to the child before birth.

Engorged Breasts This is fairly common in both female and male babies, again due to maternal hormones. The enlargement gradually disappears within days.

Eyes Sometimes the baby's tear-ducts are not yet unblocked at birth, and the eye on the blocked side (often it is only one side) waters a lot, may redden and discharge a little at times. This condition clears itself spontaneously, maybe soon after birth, or any time within the first year. Keep the eye cleansed, and you can run your fingertip very lightly down the length of the nose on the affected side — a few times a day. This form of massage may help to clear the blockage, but do it lightly. (Do it to yourself and you'll soon feel how little pressure is needed.)

Occasionally a small blood vessel breaks during delivery and you'll notice a red spot in the baby's eye. This will clear itself quite quickly.

Noses! New babies often sneeze a lot while they are adjusting to the atmosphere and light. They are noisy little people, making unpredictable sounds as they sleep, eat, and nosey around. You can use the rubber syringe to suction the baby's nose if mucous seems to be bothering her while she's asleep.

Understand that the LeBoyer bath has nothing to do

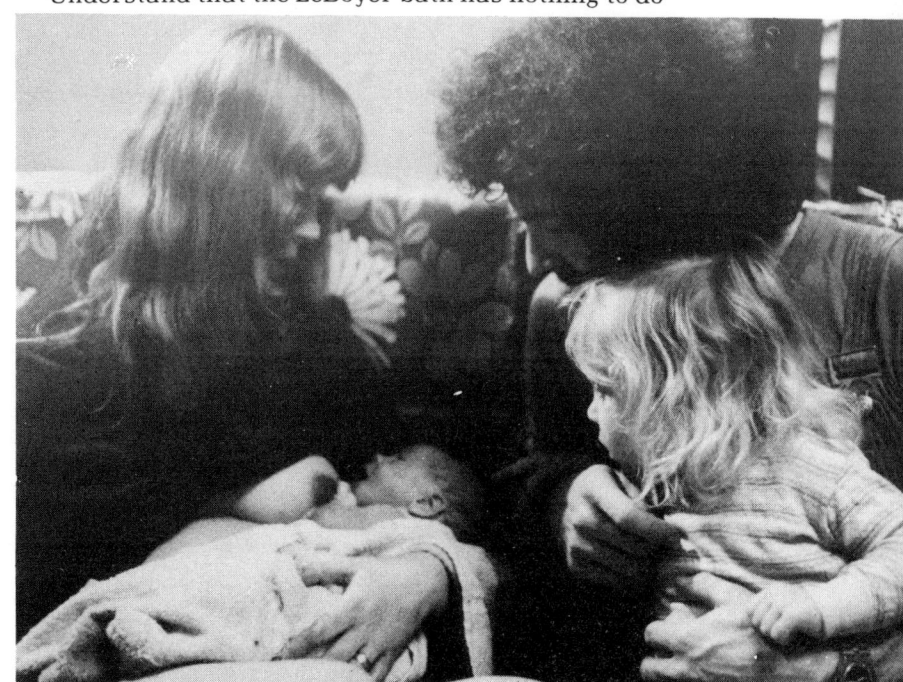

with cleansing the baby; in fact, care is taken not to remove the vernix, her own white protective cream. After the bathing, she is gently patted dry and the vernix is allowed to be fully absorbed by the skin, as it contains some vitamins, and protects the skin during its adjustment to the air. Birth without an episiotomy is very clean, but if a tear has occurred, any blood streaks can be sponged off. The baby's head should not be handled any more than is necessary for support.

The baby should pee and pass meconium within 24 hours. They very often pee at birth and this could go unnoticed if the baby is a girl — little boys usually manage to hit someone!

Sometimes the skin may dry out, particularly on the hands and feet. A gentle massage of these areas with a natural oil or lanolin will be appreciated. (Whatever Baby Oil is, it does not smell or 'feel' natural, and does not seem to mosturise the skin at all.)

Place the baby on her stomach for sleeping — mucous and milk-spills drain out safely this way., They also seem to sleep more securely on their stomachs and startle less. They have a strong instinct for survival, and will move so that they can breathe easily; they will not smother on a firm surface. Do not give a child a pillow until she begs for one (usually in their second or third year) since the longer she goes without one the better it is for her spine.

Sponge bath the baby until the cord drops off. By then she'll love to play in the bath. The skin has its own cleansing system which is destroyed by soap; besides, the baby's own smell is far more beautiful than that of Knight's Castile or any other. A daily bath is not necessary for cleaning purposes, but is a wonderful diversion, change of sensation, and a special time for one-to-one communication and pleasure (Paul always bathed our babies whenever possible; for him it was a time of closeness equal to what breastfeeding was for me.) Skin needs the stimulation of fresh air and water. While bathing the child, stimulate the scalp by massaging it with a medium-soft baby's hair-brush. This is usually enough to prevent the build up of flakey skin and cradle-cap. Don't be afraid of the 'soft-spot' — the brain is well protected by tough membranes and skin.

Babies are quite individual when it comes to crying. Some cry often, others hardly at all. The frequency should not be a bother if you consider that she has only one way to express any number of things; hunger, discomfort, the need for company, for stimulation; in protest against too much stimulation, harsh lights, unusual noise, wind cramps, and more. What is important is that she be answered and appeased. They are generally pretty easy to please, and you can soon discern her needs without conscious reflection. Every time you answer a cry (even the hard-to-figure-out ones), the baby receives a positive impression which ultimately provides the child with security and the encouragement to begin his path to independence.

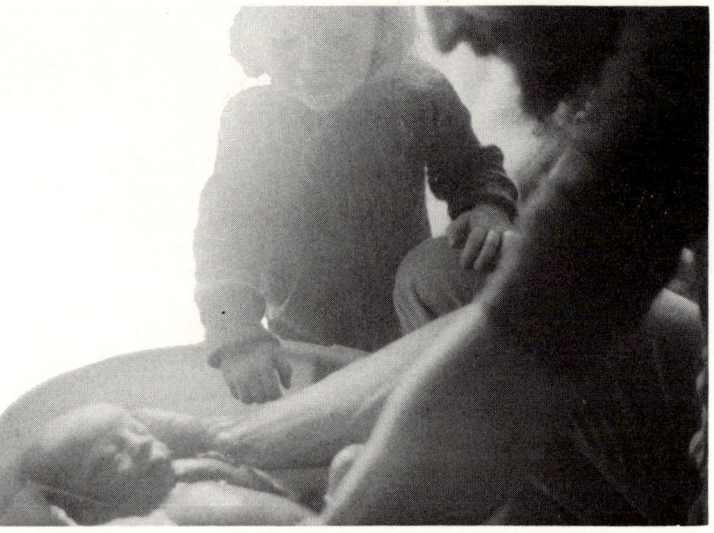

Paul and Heidi with Galen

Children at Birth

When older children attend the birth of their new sister or brother, there is no separation from the parents and no detachment from the event. Their adjustment is enhanced in much the same way as the father's is when he is fully involved. Too often, this is only possible if homebirth is chosen — a common reason for the rejection of hospital services.

The child is naturally accepting when there is no separation or alienation, and when there is no mystery. Young children who are separated from the birth often view the baby as something they'd just as soon do without and wish the baby to wherever it came from. Too often, despite the preparations, they believe the baby comes from the hospital, not from the mother. There is no sense of affinity with the new child, just resentment at the way he changes things.

When children are at birth there is no mystery, no unknown place. They are aware of the baby's presence within the mother and at birth they see it emerge from her body; that this baby is part of the family is unquestioned. All through labour, the brother or sister has watched anxious at Mummy working so hard, then relaxes and chatters when Mummy's face relaxes and stops 'breathing funny'. Perhaps the child helped by getting a cold drink, a damp cloth, or another pillow; perhaps he just held Mummy's hand and 'pushed too'.

Whatever his level of involvement, the sibling shared the work, the pain, the relief, the love — he saw his own birth. He understands life through living it. Galen's birth gave Heidi a sudden understanding of her own birth story, and she realised her own value as

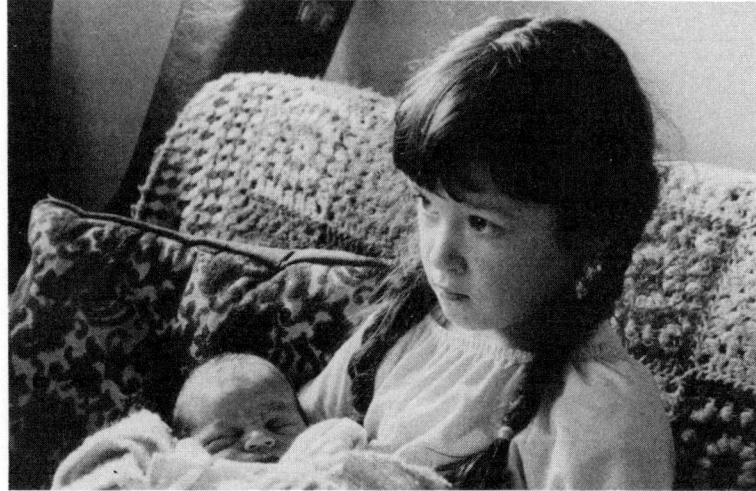

Michelle and Matthew

a wanted, welcomed, deeply loved and important member of our family. Since then her sense of origin and identity have become very strong and satisfying for her.

We know about maternal-infant bonding; we're learning about paternal-infant bonding; of course a child 'bonds' at the birth of his brother or sister! — at a homebirth, everyone does! They don't separate themselves from the new baby with white gowns, foolish face-masks, rubber gloves and a 'professional manner'. At home, people can laugh and cry, touch, stroke, cuddle and kiss a baby with true adoration and affection. The baby, free from harsh lights, silver nitrate, trolleys, scales and other mechanical

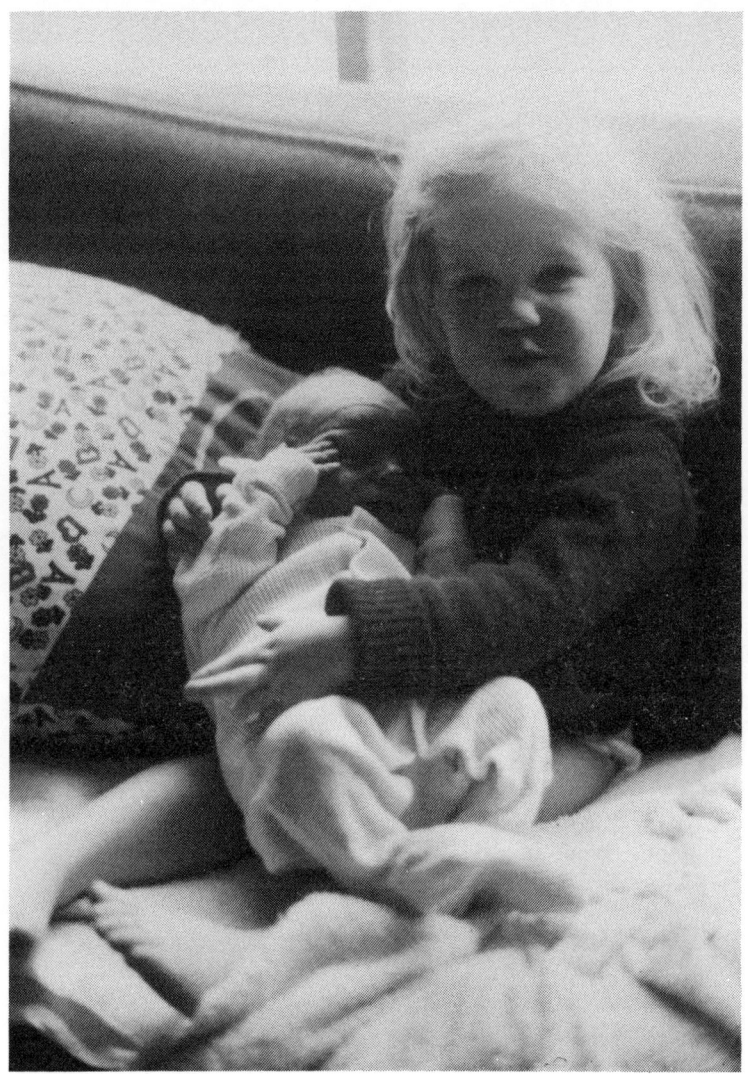

monsters, cannot help but relax, look about, reach out and 'bond' with everybody. It is a wondrous merging of bodies and spirits so strong it seems visible, physical, and measurable. (Considering the demands that the little one can put on the various members of the family over the next 12 months, it seems like a very good system).

Our children will fight and squabble superficially, but we have never had anything approaching 'sibling rivalry'. There is a visible bond between then, a need for each other and a depth of sharing that surprises us. It seems automatic as we have never asked for it. I feel that the benefits of such a shared birth go far beyond our hopes and expectations, into realms we could never have forseen.

Holistic philosophy, psychotherapy, social services, and alternative education systems represent some of the efforts to restore the life of man to one meaningful whole, balanced and natural. The need for such corrective systems would be lessened if birth returned home, if sex was not 'dirty' and therefore birth not a shameful secret. The consequences of a father attending his child's birth, a child watching his brother's birth, are likely to reflect in a social sanity that is less violent, less alienated, less materialistic — a comfortable world where a man loves his family more than his job, where a child *knows* where he came from and where he belongs.

Breastfeeding

Breastfeeding is essential to homebirth; it is the only natural conclusion. Lactation is an important period in a woman's reproductive cycle. The sucking of the newborn soon after birth causes hormones to be released which cause the placenta to separate and the uterus to contract strongly and thus prevent bleeding. It is also an important part of the bonding process.

Breastfeeding can be established very easily following a homebirth; you just flow into it. Never being separated from the child, you retain an instinctive perception of her needs. You have your own atmosphere, no imposed schedules, no medical fuss and no contradiction. Your baby will be undrugged, probably eager to nurse, and your milk will come in early. If, during pregnancy, you toughened your nipples by exposing them to sunlight and the gentle friction of clothing, you will reap the benefits now. (Inverted or flat nipples should have been drawn out and rolled or sucked daily during pregnancy, and are not a hindrance to successful nursing.) Overly protected nipples can get pretty sore quickly.

From birth on, it is best to let the baby suck as much as she wants. At some point in the first few days your nipples will feel tender from all the unaccustomed sucking — this has to be gone through as the final part of the toughening process. Cutting down on nursing time too drastically tends to prolong the tenderness and getting overly full of milk in between feeds adds to the discomfort. It is best to hang in there and get it over with — it is only a temporary problem. If one nipple is more comfortable than the other, nurse on that one first as the baby sucks more vigorously to begin with. Switch her to the other breast before she is too content to nurse any more.

Choose carefully what you apply to your nipples. You want to stop them from drying and cracking, but keeping them too soft with creams will prevent them

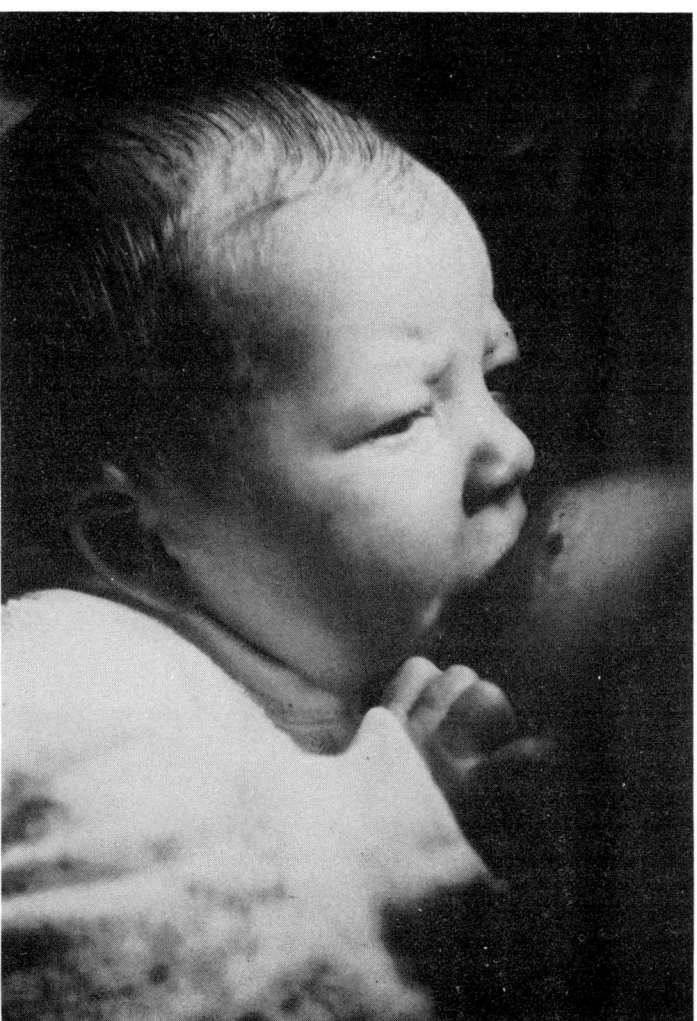

from toughening. Wash them just once or twice a day with clean water — not sterilised water. The nipples have their own cleansing system which is destroyed by soap (soap also has a drying action). After each nursing, allow the nipples to air-dry if possible before clothing yourself again. When nipples are tender, you could apply a little Vitamin A and D ointment, or some hydrous lanolin. These creams will be usefully absorbed; others tend to clog the pores. While nipples are toughening, small sucking blisters commonly occur, only to disappear again shortly. Tender nipples, uterine cramps and strange new feelings of a strong "let-down" reflex will occur each time the baby nurses over the third, fourth and fifth days. After that, apart from the "let-down" reflex which you quickly get used to, the discomforts suddenly disappear.

While establishing your milk supply, demand feeding is the best idea. Later on, when you know each other well, and baby knows that when hunger hurts she will be fed, you can try to regulate feeds a little more. After the six week growth spurt, many babies establish routines of their own which may be entirely satisfactory to you both. At various times the baby will temporarily break these routines, as subsequent growth spurts increase her nutritional requirements. She will fuss for extra feeds for 24 hours or so, during which time your body will respond and produce more milk. Then all will go back to a more normal pattern — until the next spurt.

New babies average 6 to 8 nursings each 24 hours. Some nurse in a very businesslike manner, others in a leisurely, slow or sleepy fashion. Babies have a need to suck beyond their need for milk, and often remain latched on to the breast after their hunger is satisfied. It is fine to let this happen as the baby does not overfeed by doing so. At the beginning of a feed, the milk is rich and creamy; at the end it becomes quite thin and watery. Breast milk is designed to satisfy both hunger and thirst, and the baby controls this by stopping when his needs of the moment are satisfied. Studies have been made that show some animals have very rich milk with a high fat and protein content; these animals nurse their young as little as twice a day. In contrast, animals with a low fat and protein content nurse their young almost continuously. Human milk has a low concentration of protein and is fully digested within two hours, so it is reasonable for a babe to be hungry this often. This explains the need for night feedings, although many babies do begin to sleep long stretches at night while still very young; others like to nurse at night until they wean. Within each family, every child will do it differently. Each mother and child will flow into the rhythm which works to their mutual advantage.

Babes nursing six to eight times a day do not need to be given water as well. Even throughout the hot summer days, this is enough to keep them hydrated. If you are getting at least six wet diapers to wash each day, and the urine is pale and clear, the baby is getting enough fluid. If, on the odd super-hot day, you wish to

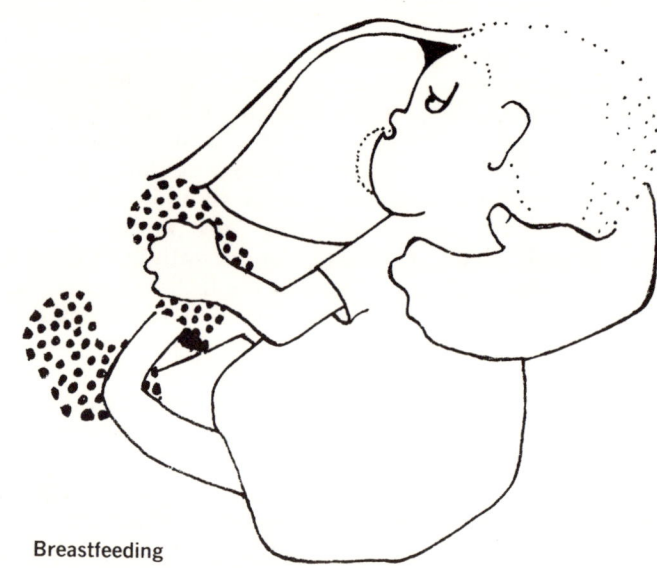

Breastfeeding

give your child water, boil it first if she is under six months old. Give it to her at room temperature, or cool, but not chilled. *Do not be tempted to sweeten it* — anything that isn't milk will cause her face to screw up distastefully at first. One of the biggest advantages of breastfeeding is that you do not foster a craving for sugar in your child, so don't blow it with sweetened water — they get to like it fine unsweetened, anyway. (Taste sweet water yourself — it's quite ikky and not at all refreshing.)

All babies spit up, some occasionally, some after every feed; this is just overflow milk. Most babies vomit occasionally, too, emptying their stomachs in the process. If it happens persistently, take the child for a check-up to find out why.

Some women are able to nurse comfortably wherever they are. If you are a person that needs privacy to relax, go right ahead and make sure you get it. Where friends or other family members are not supportive, to quietly and unobtrusively do it your way is the best answer. While breastfeeding, the most important relationship is between you and your child.

If you make an impression on other people at all, it is your calm, self-confidence that will do it; constantly defending yourself and allowing others to upset you, does no-one any good. Above all, don't accept unqualified opinions as sound advice. No-one else can tell you that you don't have enough milk, or you should be giving your child iron or whatever else. For advice, listen only to other women who have successfully. breastfed, or to someone involved in the La Leche League. Doctors are probably not knowledgeful advisors (with a few exceptions) in that they are "inexperienced", biased by the attitudes of their own wives or mothers, and often give you blatant misinformation peddled to them by representatives of 'formula' or drug manufacturers.

Being able to associate with other nursing mothers is a huge advantage. It makes you feel more normal if you live in a society that does not take breastfeeding seriously. It helps to see other women who are similarly sensitive to their babies, and to see other babies thriving wonderfully on the kind of care you want to give your child.

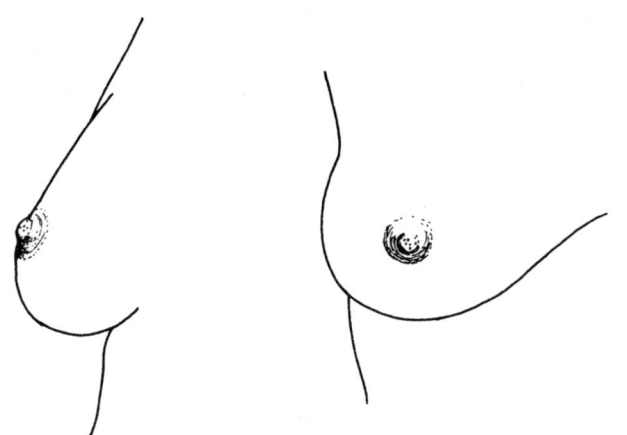

Fig.1 Non-pregnant breast

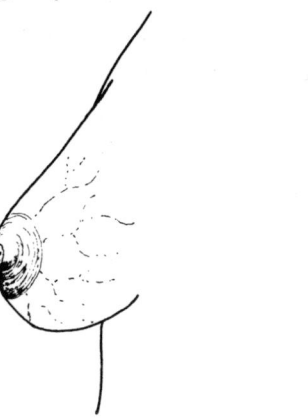

Fig.2 Lactating breast

Breast Changes

Breastmilk is nutritionally advantageous to a child for the first nine months. Beyond this, her nutritional requirements expand to include other sources of food and fluid, although nursing can continue to be a pleasure for both mother and child. The benefits to a child when she is ill or in need of special comforting and security continue indefinitely. Most children become interested in other foods at about six months of age; by 9 to 12 months, breastmilk is the supplement, but still supplying important protein, usable iron, vitamins and minerals, and filling psychological needs. When to wean is an individual decision. As the child gradually weans, the menstrual cycle returns, and with it a lessening of the mother/child drive. Hormonal changes at this time cause some women to desire total weaning, while others enjoy the nursing way beyond this time and leave the decision to the child.

NUTRITION DURING LACTATION

Maintain a natural, wholesome diet, increasing your protein intake to 110 grams a day. Keep up the supplements, as requirements increase rather than decrease. You can now use 3000mg of calcium a day, and extra vitamin D is needed for the calcium absorbtion, so take 2000 to 2500 IU of vitamin D daily. The B complex vitamins are now important to combat fatigue and maintain a good milk supply.

Continue with:
- 200 to 600 IU of vitamin E + 1mg of folic acid
- food sources of iron and B_{12} (liver, yeast)
- up to 1500mg of vitamin C
- 2500 IU of vitamin A

The baby's needs will thus be provided for through the breastmilk. Sunlight, whenever possible, will provide most of his vitamin D, and this will be supplemented in the breastmilk if you take vitamin D also. The iron content of breastmilk is very low, but ideally suited to the baby's absorbtion; all the iron is bound to a protein called lactoferrin, which enables virtually all of it to be used. Thus there is no need to supplement the child with additional iron once she reaches six months of age, which has been the custom until recently. She will get enough from breastmilk until her food takes over supplying this need.

PROBLEMS DURING LACTATION

Blocked Milk Duct   The nipple is the outlet for several milk ducts; if you squeeze it, milk may spurt in all directions. (A terrified mother once phoned to tell me her nipple had "more than one hole in it"! She was really relieved to learn she wasn't falling to pieces.) It is possible for one of these ducts to become blocked, and you'll have a tender, reddened spot, probably close to the aureola (the brown part surrounding the nipple) over the duct in question. There will be no other symptoms. To unclog the duct, encourage the baby to nurse frequently from that breast. In between nursings, apply hot cloths, cuddle a hot water bottle (without burning yourself), and take hot baths or showers. The duct will clear within a day or two.

Cracked Nipples   Try to avoid letting your nipples get dry enough to crack. If it happens, apply a mixture of honey and codliver oil, a combination which has great healing power. A cracked nipple may bleed, is sore and discouraging, but it will heal in a day or two. Favour the sore nipple by stopping the baby from sucking unnecessarily on it; that is, no more than is necessary to empty the breast. Expose the nipple to air and sunlight. Begin feeds on the other breast to avoid the most vigorous sucking on the sore nipple. Change your nursing position frequently to spread the stress. Most commercial creams are expensive and of dubious value; applying both comfrey and vitamin E is more likely to speed the healing.

Mastitis   This occurs when a duct becomes blocked, and stasis sets in. Milk builds up in that section of the breast and the mother will feel a hot, tender, reddened area and will feel sick and feverish (flu-like) as the infection develops.

As for a blocked duct, it is important to get the milk flowing through the blocked area again. Use hot compresses and nurse the baby frequently on the affected side. Nurse the baby as often as she will oblige; *do not* stop nursing as this only increases the milk back-up and then you will risk having an abscess form. A breast abscess is a painful, horrible experience, and is avoidable if you follow the cardinal rule: do not quit nursing on that side, no matter who may advise it (many doctors still do). Nurse twice as often if possible. At the first sign of breast tenderness, it is wise to begin immediately on a treatment of garlic, extra vitamin C, calcium and vitamin A as a precaution against infection. Mastitis will clear up in a couple of days.

Prevention: avoid getting run-down or over-tired as this is the usual cause. A duct may also get blocked from a too tight bra, or from sleeping too heavily on a breast.

Tuberculosis and Whooping Cough are the only infectious diseases which might cause a mother to stop breastfeeding her baby; she can nurse through all other infectious diseases. The baby develops, through her, an immunity to the diseases. When a mother becomes feverish, her milk supply diminishes temporarily, but gets back to normal in a day or two.

Other contra-indications to nursing are rare. A debilitating disease which really saps the mother's energy may be one reason; another could be a mother's absolute need to take a drug which could be harmful to the baby, e.g. drugs to control epilepsy.

SUDDEN INFANT DEATH SYNDROME

This is the subject of increasing research, although nothing conclusive has been determined yet.

One theory holds that it may be the result of a traumatic birth, and subsequent treatment which is not sufficiently sensitive to the child's needs — the child loses the will to live. This is most poignantly demonstrated by the number of institutionalised children who either die or become retarded through lack of security and stimulation.

Smothering, respiratory failure from possible allergies, sudden drop in blood-sugar levels, are other proffered reasons.

SIDS seems to occur more often among formula-fed babies than breastfed babies. Demand breastfeeding ensures that dangerous drops in the baby's blood-sugar level do not occur, while the touching, familiar

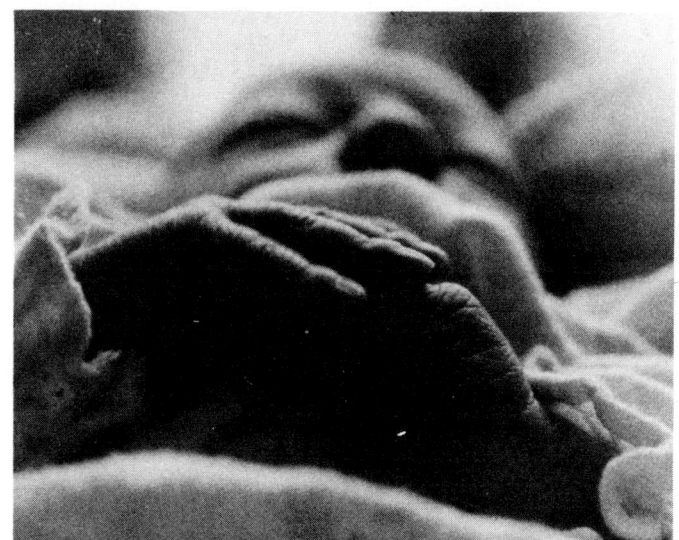

The Newborn

mother-smell, and eye-to-eye contact inevitable in breastfeeding provides the ongoing security so necessary for survival.

Dr Derrick Lonsdale, a pediatrition at the world-renowned Cleveland Clinic, has found that a Thiamine (vitamin B) deficiency is a major factor in his research into crib deaths (*Prevention*, February, 1979). He can now identify potential victims, and finds that they have in common a major defect in energy metabolism, and a lack of certain crucial enzymes. Vitamin B is important because of its oxidative power: without it the body cannot use oxygen and sugar, and is thus deprived of two essential items necessary for survival. When this error of metabolism exists, the child most at risk is the one on a high calorie diet. With today's highly processed, high-carbohydrate foods, there is a disproportionate amount of calories taken in, compared to the vitamins and minerals which protect the oxidative process. The processing of foods destroys or removes these essential ingredients, leaving 'naked' calories which choke the body. The risk is obvious with the child fed on artificial formulas and commercial baby foods. But the breast-fed baby may also suffer thiamine deficiency through a mother's poor nutritional habits.

In the States, botulism has been discovered as the cause of some infant deaths, and is linked to the intake of honey. (*"Harrowsmith"* Dec. 1978). Honey, like all raw foods, may contain botulism spores, but they pass through the mature digestive system unnoticed. The same spores may be able to grow and produce toxins in the intestines of infants. Honey has been isolated as the culprit probably because, of all the raw foods, it is the most likely to be fed to an infant. (The spores have to be heated to 248°F to be destroyed, so pasteurised honey is no safer than raw honey.) It would seem wise to avoid giving honey to infants in their first year, as the oldest infant to die from botulism traced to honey was eight months old.

Closer to home, Australian research has substantiated the dangers of the refined, high-carbohydrate diet, and also linked SIDS to vaccination injury and insufficient vitamin C (see Chapter: *Immunisation and Childhood Diseases*, for further details).

Clearly, no single cause can be identified. We can only apply all the current research data to the carefully assessed diets of both the mother and baby.

— Resources —

"Drugs in Breast Milk, A Consumer Guide". Birth & The Family Journal.
This reprint is available from the ICEA Book Centre.

La Leche League International, Inc. 9616 Minneapolis Ave., Franklin Park, Ill. 60131, USA.
They have a comprehensive paper on drugs in breast milk, and all other information you might need. If there is no L.L. group in your area, write to this address or call (312)455-7730 Illinois, USA.

La Leche League, New Zealand Co-Ordinator; P.O. Box 242, Pukekohe, South Auckland.

— Reading —

Pryor, Karen.   **Nursing Your Baby**
Helpful, enjoyable reading.

Ewey, Donna & Roger   **Preparation for Breastfeeding.**

Kipley, Sheila.   **Breastfeeding & Natural Child Spacing.**
This has a particularly sensitive approach to mothering.

Raphael, Dana   **The Tender Gift: Breastfeeding.**

NOTE: **Spiritual Midwifery** while recommended elsewhere, does contain several inaccuracies relating to breastfeeding.

Discovering Childbirth and the Joy of Breastfeeding
Pauline O'Brien

Immunisation and Childhood Illnesses

If you intend to vaccinate your child and are breast-feeding, do not begin the series until the child is six months old. Prior to this, the child is protected by antibodies in the breastmilk against all the diseases the mother has had or been vaccinated against. These same antibodies will work against vaccines and counter them before the child's body has produced its own antibodies; the child remains unprotected by the vaccinations. After six months, the mother's antibodies are less likely to dominate.

Some people consider vaccines an insult to the body and against nature. If you decide, for whatever reason not to vaccinate, added responsibility is upon you; you have to know that at all times your children are in proper condition to handle disease and build up resistance. This is impossible on a junk-food diet, but is possible if good food is the rule.

In order to become a healthy adult, a child's body must build up healthy resistances. Childhood illnesses should be considered as natural cleansing processes; that is, getting sick is necessary and desirable. But strung-out illnesses and the variety of complications we see today are not necessary or desirable. This is what happens when a child is not equipped to resist disease to begin with, and is then not helped by the treatment given.

Polio   Since polio vaccine has been in use, the disease is no longer a problem, but bone and muscle damage is a fairly common side effect of the vaccination.

The tonsils play an important role both in preventing polio and in modifying the intensity of the disease. Many victims of fashionable tonsilectomies went on to become paralysed victims of severe poliomyelitis in the '30s and '40s. Paralysis is rare where tonsils have not been removed.

Fever, vomiting and flu-like symptoms precede identification of polio virus. Dr. Mayerhofer, a German biologist, states that polio can only be contracted after an episode of intestinal catarrh (i.e. irritation or inflam-

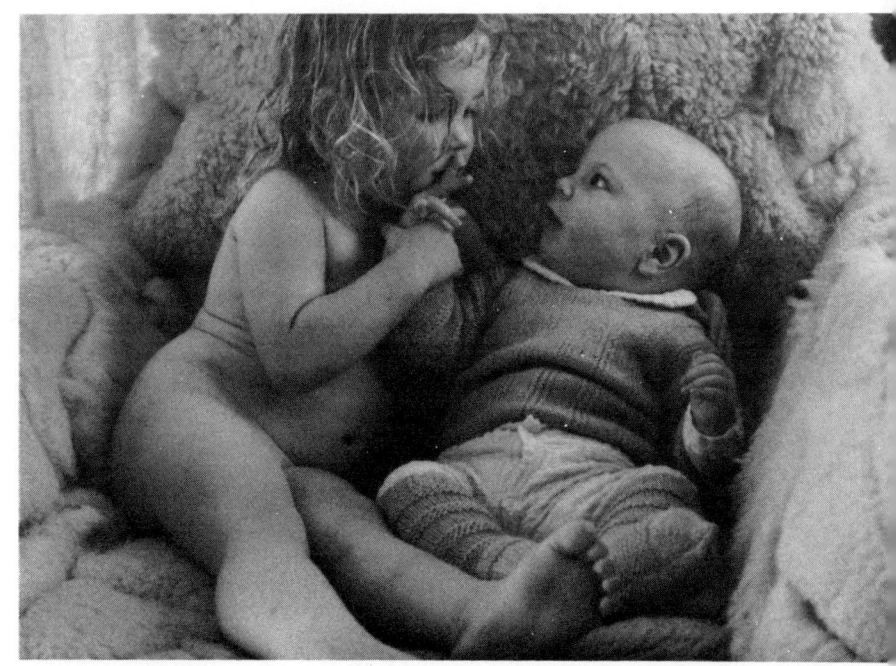

mation of the digestive tract, as in 'flu). He used garlic to prevent intestinal catarrh, and thus prevented his patients from contracting polio. In another experiment with Swedish school children in a polio outbreak area, no children given garlic tablets (1204 children took two tablets daily) contracted polio, while 67 children whose parents refused permission for the treatment did get polio.

The antibiotic properties of garlic are also fully effective (and sometimes superior to penicillin) against rheumatic fever, tuberculosis, typhoid, cholera, scarlet fever, diptheria and whooping cough.

Smallpox   The hazards of smallpox vaccinations are now recognised, and this vaccination is no longer mandatory.

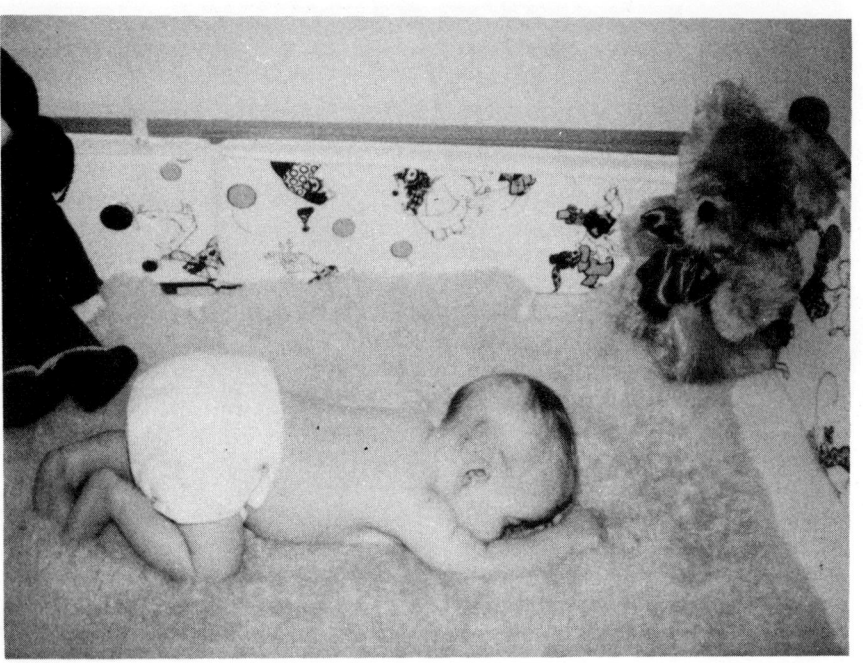

Diptheria   When diptheria vaccinations became available, it was found there was a decline in death rate among unimmunised people as well as those vaccinated, in about the same proportions. The British Ministry of Health stated that other factors seemed to be more relevant; improved personal hygiene, more care over water supplies, and better drainage and sewer systems. Due to steadily improving sanitation, diptheria was strongly on the decline *before* immunisation was begun.

Clinical research by Australian doctors Archivides Kalokerinos and Glen Dettman has enlightened us to the dangers of low vitamin C intake. Refined foods, high carbohydrate foods, and frozen foods may contain little or no vitamin C, and this vitamin, in small amounts, is oxidised so rapidly that it is of little benefit. They explain that vitamin C is a liver metabolite, needed for the proper functioning of almost all chemical processes in the body, and is an essential factor in our body's defence system. They do not support immunisation campaigns; they see vaccinations as an immunological insult which actually lowers resistance to disease. They have recorded adult deaths following vaccinations. They have also found that infants with low vitamin C content in their bodies are likely to die shortly after receiving immunisation shots — deaths which pathologists will attribute to heart failure, but which are highly likely to be 'crib deaths' resulting from the baby's inability to manufacture the necessary antibodies to cope with the onslaught of introduced infection. Without vitamin C, the body is at risk both from naturally acquired infections and from immunisation shots. These doctors have had complete success in preventing crib deaths and post-immunisation deaths with their Vitamin C Therapy.

If you decide to have your children vaccinated, your doctor should make you aware of all the risks involved — you must be giving your *informed consent*. Before each vaccination, make sure your child is fed a strictly natural, nutritious diet to supply the vitamins and minerals needed for the body to be able to form antibodies: namely, vitamins A, B complex, C and Calcium. The diet should be high in protein. Adhere strictly to this for a few days after the vaccination. Extra vitamin C is important afterwards to protect against "vaccination injury" — that is, the fever, and possible damaging side effects of the vaccines. Do not ignore any resulting fever or illness as an expected response; while most children recover satisfactorily, you cannot ignore the large number of children who suffer damage of some kind, ranging from mild to severe, permanent, or the occasional death. For fevers, give vitamin A and massive doses of vitamin C.

Doctors Kalokerinos and Dettman recommend that pregnant and lactating women take up to 15,000mgm daily. Children should receive 1000mgm a day for each year of age up to the age of ten (e.g. 3,000mgm a day for three-year-olds). Sick infants should receive even more.

A clean, healthy body, achieved by natural, unrefined foods, exercise and food supplements as necessary, has a high potential resistance to all infection. If, at the first sign of illness, the child is given the additional quantities of nutrients her body needs to fight the disease and cope with the added stress, the child has a much healthier method of resistance. Parents who have tried it, report that illnesses are shorter-lived than normal, and complications or secondary diseases are rare.

Use garlic as an antibiotic if you suspect an ear, nose, throat, chest or gasto-intestinal infection. Acidophillus is an antibiotic also effective against both intestinal infections and genito-urinary infections. Include extra doses of vitamin C in all instances. Our young children chew these supplements as readily as others enjoy candies.

I must repeat this: if you ever give your children prescribed antibiotics, be sure to give them acidophillus tablets or yoghurt, and extra vitamin C throughout and beyond the course to avoid damaging side-effects and to replace the healthy intestinal bacteria which will be destroyed.

- Recommended Reading -

Stone, Irwin.   **The Healing Factor**

Parenting

The new baby, a tiny creature with no knowledge of the Queen's English, can fill a day so full that there is hardly any time to go to the bathroom, let alone read books on Parenting. Yet at some point I think we all need to turn to books, for children specialise in blowing preconceived theories to smithereens and presenting us with previously unimagined situations. The next problem, then, is where to start; so much is written on the subject of parenting and so much of it is contradictory.

As parents, your vulnerability is not helped by the current onslaught of 'prescription' literature — books which provide us with hypothetical circumstances and a choice of processed, pre-packaged answers which will 'fit' providing our children create a similar scene. There are even books which teach us to speak 'Childrenese'!

Fortunately, there are authors who still believe that people cannot be so easily categorised, and who appreciate the value of imagination, humour, and human fallibility. They boost our confidence by granting us our weaknesses and imperfections, stressing change through learning and growing with our children, making us feel that ordinary people *can* parent, and putting our goof-ups into a healthy, shameless, human perspective.

The most useful information provides us with insight and understanding of what our children are going through. With adult values being so different to childhood needs, we must learn what infants and children experience, and how it is important to their growth and development. Armed with this knowledge, we can then figure out how to handle things as they occur. We do not need Parenting Prescriptions; they destroy our individuality and tend to focus our sights on success or failure, instead of the joys and challenges of every fresh, new day. Understanding and acceptance of our own individuality will assist the child to pass through each stage with his needs fulfilled, his magic intact.

Whatever philosphy we choose, the most important thing is to be able to sift out advice that feels good, and disregard anything that would hurt in practice. With the best intentions in the world, leading child specialists are still encouraging us to do depressing, bond-damaging things like letting children 'cry it out' or forcing an infant who needs company to sleep alone at night. Obviously this is not good advice if the baby is

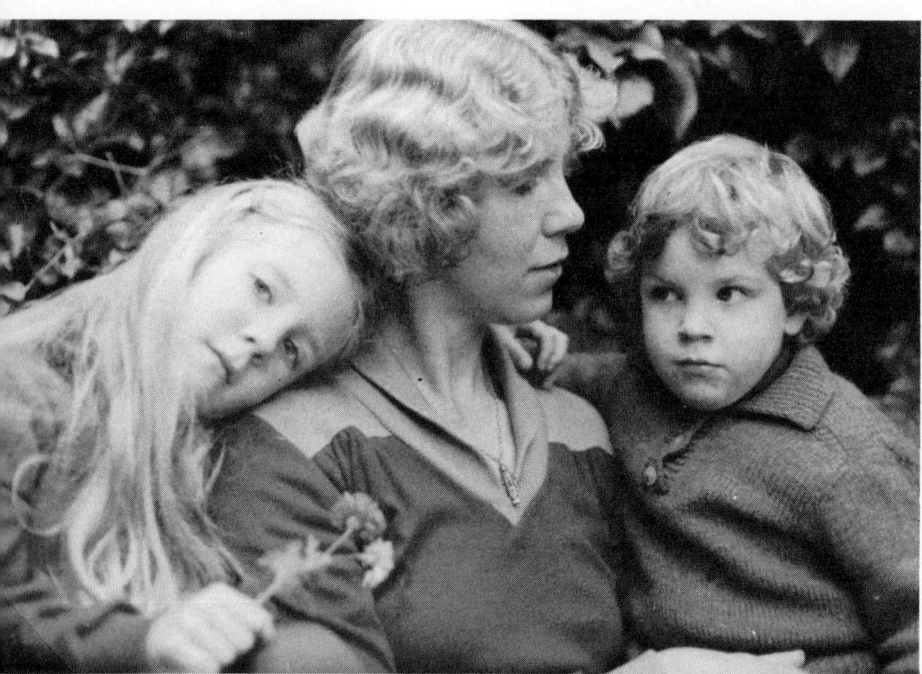

Ingrid with Heidi and Galen

screaming in one room and you are sobbing quietly in another.

A major destroyer of confidence is the typical birth experience. A woman is stripped of her dignity and ability, delivered of a child by a doctor and his tools because he does not expect her to be able to do it alone; a man is possibly 'allowed' to witness the birth of his child, or he may be banished from the scene as a possible source of infection. The child they take home is a relative stranger; a huge negative experience separates the reality of the child from the joyful anticipation of pregnancy. The parents must struggle to get their individual selves together again, and find it very hard to cope with the new dimension of their family. But we are learning that one of the effects of a natural, shared, family birth is a great boost of self-confidence, a wonderful enhancing of one's self-image. Homebirth bonding ensures an even flow into the daily responsibilities; it does not eliminate problems, but it does change them. Men who are active participants become proudly involved in their child's rearing and wellbeing and display many 'motherly' instincts. The child is no stranger, no intruder. Challenges are met by a solid, family team, charged by the shared bonding experience of the child's birth.

Being deeply bonded to your child, and friendly with your own instincts, gives you fewer decisions to make in child rearing. A major reason for birthing outside of the hospital is to remain in constant physical and spiritual contact with the child. Thus you are less likely to get confused about conforming to useless social customs when the child no longer qualifies for newborn considerations. The fewer traumatic socialising pressures the child experiences, the fewer 'expected' problems you'll face. The child will socialise himself when he is ready; even the experts agree that the child desires to please those he loves, and struggles to copy his parents, to become part of the things they do. Being an acceptable part of the family is extrememly important to every child. Realising this, premature socialising seems foolish and likely to **undermine** his growth. The unpressured child strives to become independent and sociable quite freely as soon as he is able. It is the pressured child that has all the eating problems, sleeping problems, training problems, rivalry problems. That family strives to endure and is shaken by the daily traumas; by the time the child should be eager and able to cope with milestones in natural progression, his self-esteem is low and he already feels incapable and unacceptable.

Security is not acquired quickly nor acquired intellectually; it is the end result of a fairly long, demanding period. When his demands are met constantly over many months, the child grows certain, deep within himself, that he is loved and cared for, that he is valuable and his needs are worthy. The constant demands of the infant and young child are not outrageous when we realise that any new relationship begins in essentially the same way, whether in childhood or adult life. Romance follows quite the same pattern of uncertainty, trial and dependence, which grows into security, trust and independence as the relationship develops. Unfortunately, a child was not

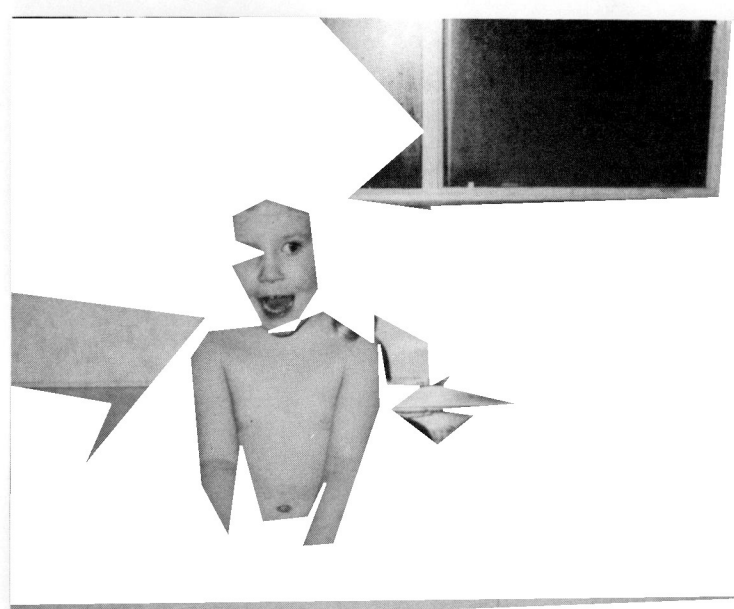

(until recently) meant to have needs, or especially to change a relationship. We were taught that children should be "seen and not heard" and that parents must preserve their privacy at all costs. So some of us are still pioneers in a new era of child raising, where we admit that children *do* change us, children *do* have rights, and although they are younger and smaller, they are in no way inferior. If we can see our children's magic, we can humbly admit they are intrinsically superior; yet it is up to us to guide these vulnerable spirits.

THE COUPLE BECOMES A FAMILY

The man's willing involvement in child raising is essential when we contemplate the changes a couple undergoes after the first child is born. There is a time of difficult adjustment for all couples, a period where parents really need the joys and togetherness of a shared birth for their own survival. If pregnancy follows a lengthy relationship, suddenly being three after a long time of being two is drastically different, but at least the couple have their own relationship well established. If the relationship has been brief, the child will break into the couple's period of learning about themselves and each other.

While nursing, the woman's hormones cause her to feel a very strong mother/infant drive. Breastfeeding is well recognised as being sexually pleasurable for most women — and fortunately so, for it is also a time-consuming, binding commitment. While some women do maintain their man/woman drive during this time, there is a lot of disappointment, guilt and resentment from couples who find their sexual activity has dwindled drastically. After the freedom of a childless relationship, the change is frightening. For about six months after the birth, the mother tends to lose sight of herself altogether; in the process of adjustment, she has little time to see herself as an individual.

Men frequently feel 'left-out'. The new mother might need considerable 'working on' to arouse sexual interest, and if the baby should cry at that delicate time, baby comes first. This displaced centre of attention is very difficult for the husband to accept; he no longer comes first and his sexual contribution to the relationship seems to be less necessary. Difficult as it may be, he must first of all understand the cause of this change in his wife's attitude — the hormonal changes brought on by lactation, and secondly, he must sublimate much of his sexual drive to serve the family in a new way, spending all the time and energy he has caring for and enjoying his wee babe, and helping his lady with the dreary reality of washing diapers and preparing meals — breastfeeding consumes a great deal of her energy and she has little left to keep the orderly house he is accustomed to.

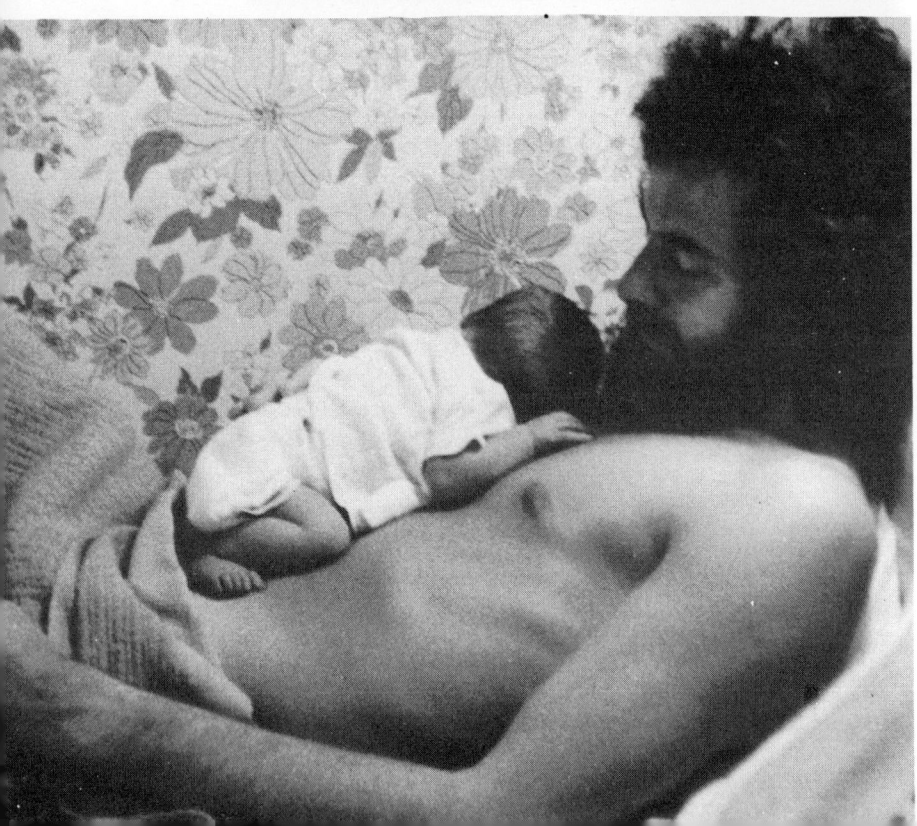

Paul and newborn Heidi

After about six months, the mother seems able to become her own person again and the relationship is more comfortable. The discouraging changes are now easier to understand and get into perspective. As the child begins to take other nourishment, and spends a few more moments playing away from his mother's skirts, the woman is more likely to feel energy and desire for her mate's relationship. Raven Lang suggests that normal sexual drive returns with the re-establishment of ovulation; this fits the experience of many women.

After a birth, it is usually a few weeks before normal vaginal lubrication returns. Some women experience an uncomfortable dryness for several weeks, and so a lubricating jelly should be used to preclude an added deterrent to sexual enjoyment.

Fortunately, after subsequent babies, the amount of understanding is far greater, and the adjustments far fewer. To make these adjustments easier in the first place, it pays to do whatever seems sensible and to ignore contrary advice. When our daughter was a few months old, we finally realised that trying to keep her separate from us was ridiculous. She hated her crib, and would wake from the deepest sleep whenever Paul and I found time to be together for a while. We eventually discovered that our privacy depended not on whether she was asleep but where she was asleep. Tucked into a corner of our bed, she would sleep soundly, giving us all the time together we could possibly want. We had wasted much valuable time trying to preserve our privacy and give her hers. But we'd been doing it by exclusion, not inclusion, and it didn't work. Once we had heard her properly, and realised that a baby's needs differ greatly from what society dictates, our lives became much easier and a lot more satisfying.

Our bed is now a wall-to-wall mattress. Our two children sleep together, beside us. Most children, even as infants, express a need to sleep with their parents; humans are the only species which force separation upon babies at bedtime. The ruses to coerce a child to accept sleeping alone are time-consuming and elaborate, and generally involve some form of mother-substitutes, like toys, special blanket, pacifiers (the ultimate insult to a child's dignity), or even recorded

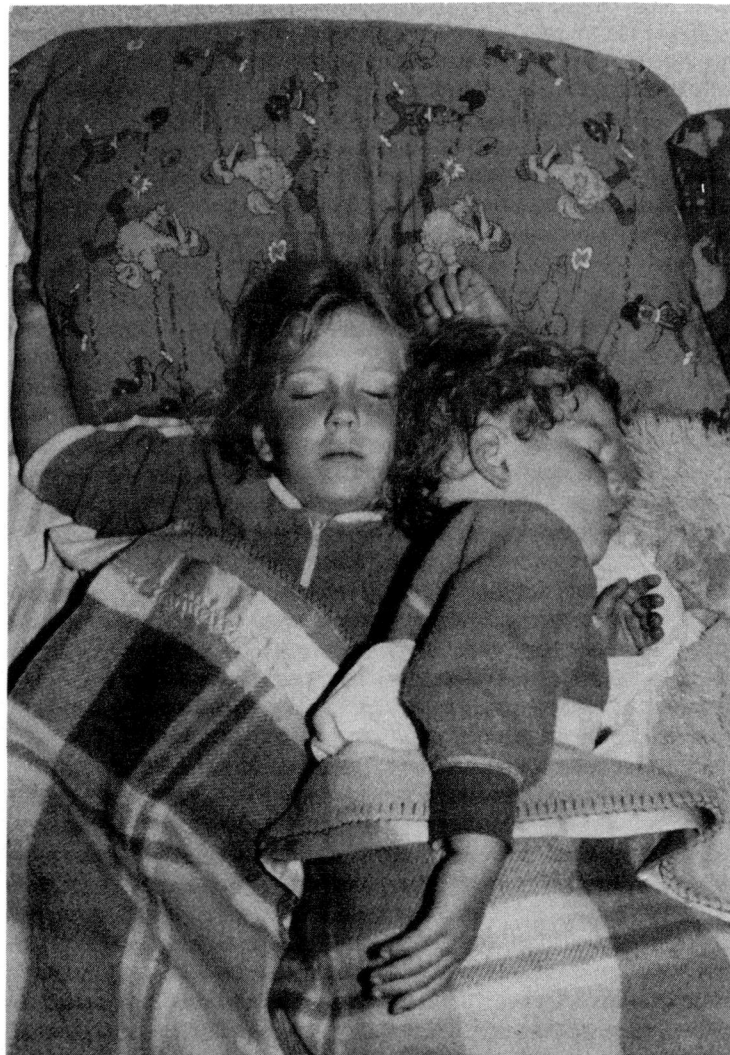

heart sounds. None of the child authorities are able to admit that the child is expressing an instinctive need, even though 100% of all infants should choose to sleep with company if so allowed. But they do go on to offer similarly elaborate cures for nightly procrastinations, crying, fear of the dark, nightmares, prolonged bed-wetting and more. The several dark hours of warm security and togetherness each night promotes the adventurous independence of our two little ones by day. I am convinced that the hours of "security-recharge" at night are essential to their personal growth. I wonder how many children are slow developers because they loose sleep, and consume energy on sleep-related problems, energy which should be used on normal development and growth.

Our days begin with the joyful, childish greeting of the new day, and end as we go gladly to bed to join our sleeping beauties. The time will come when they will want to sleep further apart from us. We don't look forward to that, but we'll let them go, grateful to have ignored well-meaning advice and treasuring these few brief years of mutually benefiting closeness.

This nightly closeness can play a large part in our personal growth as parents. A man cannot resent the warm, sweet-smelling babe nestled into his armpit, the same child who demands his wife's attention all day long. The children who leave you drained and exhausted, desperate for sleep, are not going to call out all night from another room; they will either sleep soundly right through, or creep in close and snuggle down 'fitting just right', making you feel needed and cherished and totally in love with them.

Sleeping close to the children is comforting for the working parent(s) who fear losing touch with their children through being away during the day. Closeness at night could be just as important to the children in this instance. The nuclear family needs all the fortification it can get, and sleeping together is one excellent way.

"Family" is parents and children, growing together, profoundly affecting each other. Children force us to take stock of ourselves, and undergo personal development that might otherwise have been delayed or avoided. They smooth off the rougher edges of our ego. They give us unlimited freedom to regress when we will, to get in the sandbox and build great castles, to create marvellous Lego machines, to buy and read all the old favourite books that no childless adult would be seen reading ever again, and to once again be enchanted by the magic and mystery of Walt Disney classics.

— Reading —

Salk, Dr Lee	How to Raise a Human Being Preparing for Parenthood
Pearse, Joseph	Magical Child
Le Shan, Eda	Natural Parenthood
Janov, Dr Arthur	The Feeling Child
Fraiberg, Selma	The Magic Years
Ribble, Margaret A.	The Rights of Infants
Briggs, Dorothy Corkille	Your Child's Self-Esteem
Dinkmeyer, Dr Don and Dr Gary D McKay	
	Raising a Responsible Child

(The last two books both involve some 'prescription' but also present good background information.)

Thevenin, Tina	The Family Bed

Appendix I

PROBLEM SOLVING DURING PREGNANCY

Varicose Veins Avoid sitting with your legs crossed — this is very bad for the circulation. If your work involves a lot of sitting, get up and stretch your legs more frequently than normal. If you have to do a lot of standing, take some time during the day, or after work, to lie with your legs elevated. If varicose veins develop, you may have to wear support hose. Take 400 IU of vitamin E twice a day for two weeks, then maintain yourself on 400 IU once a day.

Anaemia Anytime your doctor checks your haemoglobin, ask him what it is and record it for yourself. If you do tend to become anaemic, see to it that your doctor investigates fully to find the cause; then treat it. If it is purely an iron deficiency anaemia, try to raise your haemoglobin count by concentrating on your diet. Include hearty doses of liver and other organ meats, eggs, fish, green vegetables, dried fruits and dessicated liver. Anaemia must be taken seriously; it becomes a considerable risk if not brought under control. There are a variety of unpleasant, debilitating symptoms and an increased liability to post-partum haemorrhage. The fetus might receive less oxygen — a major cause of brain damage — and the child will also become anaemic shortly after birth. If anaemia is a problem, Adelle Davis goes into helpful detail in *Let's Have Healthy Children*.

B_{12} and Folic Acid Anaemia Several of the B vitamins, including folic acid, are destroyed by antibiotics, sulpha drugs and arsenic (traces of which get into our fruit and vegetables). Oral contraceptives also deplete our B vitamin reserves. B_{12} occurs only in minute amounts in vegetarian food sources, and all B vitamins are almost entirely eliminated from the highly processed 'Convenience' foods.

During pregnancy, the body's need for the B vitamins, B_{12} and Folic Acid, is substantially increased; consequently, deficiencies have become more commonplace. At least one in five pregnant women are deficient in folic acid — the consequences of which are serious. Its symptoms are: tiredness, poor appetite, nausea, perhaps vomiting and diarrhoea.

More than half the women who miscarry or experience spotting during pregnancy are found deficient in folic acid. Apruptio placentae, or premature separation of the placenta — one cause of premature labour — may occur when folic acid is deficient. Deformed babies are twice as common, and cleft palate is the result of this deficiency at the time when the palate normally closes.

Brewers yeast and dessicated liver should be included in large quantities in vegetarian diets, especially during pregnancy and throughout lactation, to supply 1 to 5mg of folic acid and 15mcg B_{12}. No vitamin ever works alone; vitamin A is also important in this context. Note that many vitamin supplements do not contain any folic acid at all.

B_{12} has also been found deficient in a significant number of women suffering post-partum depression; B_{12} therapy promptly reversed the symptoms.

Toxaemia This is a condition peculiar to pregnancy, the cause of which does seem to be various nutritional deficiencies, and becoming much less common now with good prenatal care, good nutrition and diet supplements. It is characterised by oedema (fluid accumlating in the tissues), high blood pressure, albumin in the urine, plus a sudden weight gain. Untreated, headaches and visual disturbances occur, and the oedema spreads giving the face, hands and whole body, a puffy appearance. The mother will become extremely ill and suffer fatal convulsions; the baby will likely be stillborn. So be aware of the danger signs and do not hesitate to get them checked out. If you do begin to get toxic, get into Adelle Davis right away, as she offers detailed changes in the diet and additonal supplements to reverse the disorder before it becomes serious. Never attempt homebirth if the symptoms do not disappear altogether; and do not slack up on your diet once you achieve a reversal. Again, the condition is unusual on a high protein, natural food diet with sensible supplements.

High Blood Pressure   This may or may not be a sign of toxaemia; it may be the result of choline deficiency, or it may result from excessive salt intake. Take B complex to supply 100mg of choline daily and restrict your salt intake. Sometimes extra potassium will lower the blood pressure. Garlic lowers blood pressure, but don't settle for this way out without first checking for the cause of your condition.

Breech Position   A persistent breech should not be handled at home without experienced help. Occasionally, the baby can surprise you by presenting bottom first, but most often a breech is diagnosed beforehand. You can determine it by abdominal palpation; by how the baby feels to the mother and by the location of the movements; also from where the fetal heart is heard.

Dr Juliet De Sa Souza has an 80% success rate with her method of "Changing the Breech Position". Quite simply, she gets her patients to lie on a hard surface with the pelvis raised on pillows to a level of 9 to 12 inches higher than the head. This should be practiced for ten minutes, twice a day, on an empty stomach. The treatment is most effective when started at the 30th week of pregnancy and continued for at least four to six weeks, or until the baby turns. Don't do the exercise once the baby turns, or he might just turn right round again! Three-quarters of the babies turn within two or three weeks.

When the baby is breech, the fetal heart is heard loudest at the level of the umbilicus or higher. In cephalic presentation (head down) the heartbeat is heard below the umbilicus.

Transverse Presentation   This cannot be handled at home. Unless the baby turns spontaneously, or the doctor is able to effect an external version at the onset of labour, Caesarian Section may be the only alternative.

Placenta Praevia   In this condition the placenta is situated in the lower segment of the uterus, either partially or completely over the cervix. Bleeding occurs in the last three months and the condition is diagnosed. Homebirth is impossible; get expert medical attention.

Abruptio Placenta   This is a premature separation of the placenta, partially or wholly, from the wall of the uterus. There may be vaginal bleeding, or severe abdominal pain and shock from internal bleeding. Get expert help.

Rh Incompatability   The blood streams of the mother and child are not supposed to mix. You can do your best to see that they don't by strengthening your capillary system. Your diet must be natural and rich in vitamin C and bioflavanoids. Vitamin C combined with bioflavanoids in powder form is available, and should be taken liberally. Other sources of bioflavinoids are whole buckwheat, the inner layers of citrus peels, and the inner core of green pepper.

Unless this is your first pregnancy, you will have had blood Rh antibody tests done. Soon after giving birth, an Rh negative mother who gives birth to an Rh positive child is given a vaccine to destroy any of the baby's Rh cells which have spilled into her blood stream before her own immunity system is triggered to produce antibodies. This means that future pregnancies will not be endangered by the presence of Rh antibodies. This injection, Rhogam, must be given within 72 hours of delivery. (It must also be given to Rh negative mothers following an abortion or miscarriage).

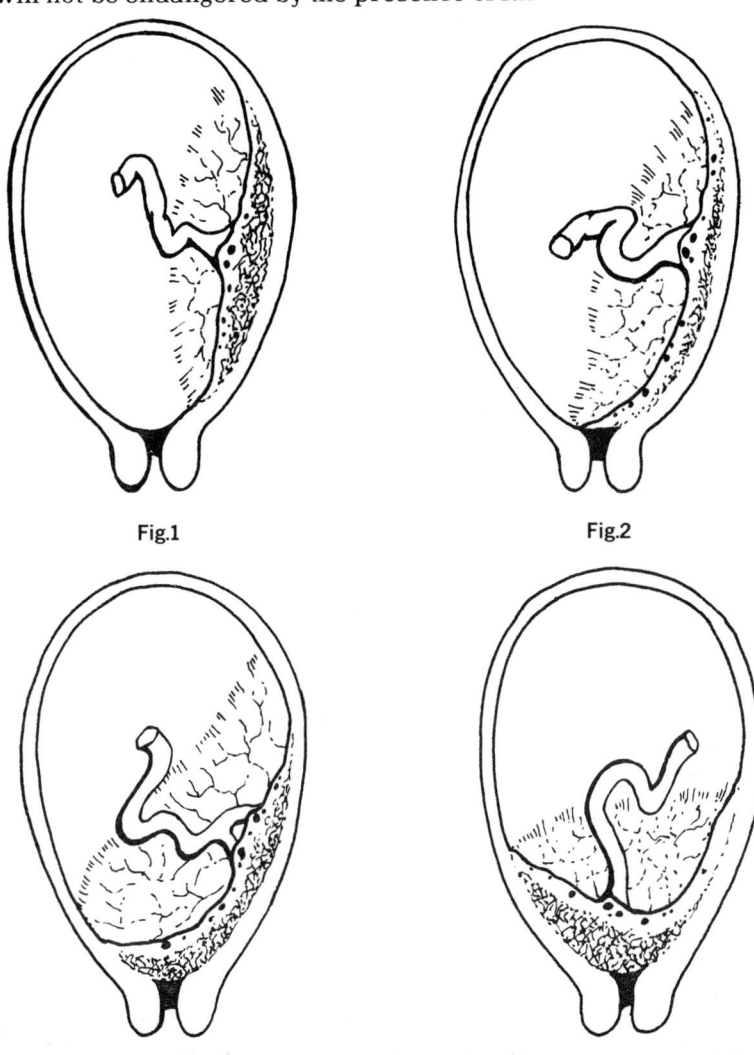

Fig.1

Fig.2

Fig.3

Fig.4

Placenta Praevia

Fig.1 Placenta abnormally low, spreads into lower segment of uterus, but not over cervix. Bleeding may occur, but birth should proceed normally.

Fig.2 Placenta covers closed cervix. Bleeding will occur from small area of placental separation as cervix dilates, but normal birth may follow.

Fig.3 and Fig.4
Placenta completely covers cervix Caesarian delivery essential.

Rash   A friend and I both experienced a brief period of itchy, unsightly rash towards the end of our second pregnancies. This seems to be due to a high hormonal level which the liver is unable to cope with. Maybe you could avoid it, or cure it, by nutritionally pampering the liver with nutrients that ease its workload. These include extra vitamin A and B complex, and up to 100g of protein a day. Garlic is a good liver tonic, and grapes especially fine liver food. Dandelion tea and raw carrot juice may be useful.

Premature Rupture of the Membranes

Amniotic fluid is produced continually, so you are never dry (a 'dry birth' is just another myth). Once the membranes rupture, there is increased risk of infection, so avoid intercourse, take showers instead of baths and be religious about hygiene. Take garlic and acidophilus as precautionary antibiotic measures. You should get medical advice, especially if you are under 37 or 38 weeks along. I know women who have refused to become hospitalised, refused the offer of an induction, and by being really alert to their bodies for any danger signs, they went on to deliver spontaneously much closer to full term than would otherwise have been likely. Sometimes a small leak in the membranes will heal itself.

DURING LABOUR

Prolonged Labour   Some labours are simply slow; sometimes contractions stop altogether for a period of time and this can happen more than once. At home where there are no deadlines to meet and you have the freedom to do what you want with no-one trying to pressure your body into a tidy, textbook pattern of labour, there should be no worry or frustration or impatience about it. You can rest, go walking, eat, or do what you want when you want. Work on the atmosphere, or any fears or tensions, if this seems to be a problem.

If you feel a need to try stimulating your labour, have a warm shower or bath (shower if the membranes have ruptured). Often after a rest or warm bath, the contractions will resume. As long as the mother feels fine and the baby shows no sign of distress, sluggish labour is not a problem requiring intervention as it will progress slowly to birth.

Preventative measures should be noted: go into labour well rested; eat to provide your body with a sustaining blood-sugar level when you first go into labour, and maintain your strength with honey-sweetened fluids and foods as you desire; alternate periods of walking with periods of rest; pee every hour. This should all prevent the mother becoming overtired.

Prolonged labour to worry about is a labour in which contractions occur regularly and are constantly demanding on the woman's energy resources — WITHOUT evident progress. After 30 to 36 hours of this kind of energy drain, a woman may quickly

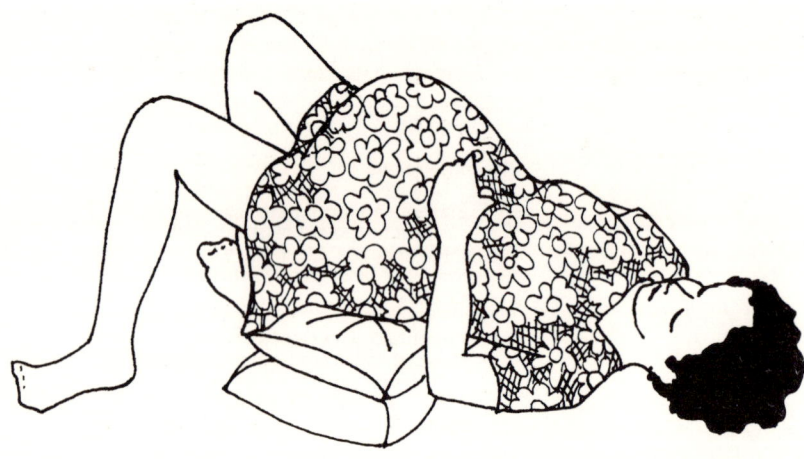

Dr. Juliet De Sa Souza's position for "Changing the Breech Position".

become exhausted; you cannot dispel anxiety at this point for something could definitely be wrong. It is possible that the baby's head is too big to pass through the pelvis, or the baby may be malpositioned and unable to turn. If either of these is suspected, medical aid should be sought. You should be in constant touch with the baby to detect signs of distress — get help immediately if this occurs.

Back Labour   Sometimes a woman feels her contractions in her back instead of her abdomen or pelvis as expected. But true back labour is very different from the usual pattern of labour. The contractions are not felt distinctly and there is no period of comfort in between them. Instead there is a constant, uncomfortable backache which intensifies as contractions peak. This labour is usually a result of the way the baby is lying — a posterior position from which he must turn in the course of labour. All good books on Prepared Childbirth illustrate and describe exercises and positions for coping with back labour; become familiar with them, as about 20% of labours are back labours. It is not a complication which threatens the outcome of labour, but it is usually a longer first stage and a harder one to handle. Incorporate some squatting into your activities, as this throws your body into the easiest position to accomplish a turn. The second stage will probably follow normal patterns.

Abnormal Maternal Signs   A woman who, for some unexpected reason, becomes ill during labour, will display any of these symptoms: she may be feverish, pale, clammy to touch, her heart may race and her pulse will be shallow and thready; she may make uncontrollable spastic movements; severe pain unrelated to the contractions may be felt; bleeding might occur; she might become extremely anxious and apprehensive; a rise in blood pressure above 140/90, or a sudden drop from the normal, is cause for alarm. Whatever the symptoms, labour would be best completed in hospital, as only a doctor would be able to diagnose the cause accurately, and the complication would justify medical intervention. It is very rare for a woman to become distressed in this manner. Possible causes could be Abruptio Placenta, or, more rarely still, the sudden onset of Eclampsia (severe toxaemia).

Fetal Distress   The baby's heart rate is your best indication of his wellbeing. You should be quite familiar with the rhythm and number of beats per minute that is normal for your baby. During labour it will not change appreciably, although during contractions the rate will slow down a little only to pick up again within 10 to 15 seconds. By listening to and counting the fetal heart during a contraction you will learn how much it decelerates.

The normal range for a fetal heart is from 120 to 160 beats per minute, the average being 140. For the sake of assessing the baby's wellbeing and detecting signs of distress, count in the intervals between contractions, not during or right after one. Distress is evidenced by a marked slowing or irregularity of the fetal heart tones; an increase of 20 beats a minute is alarming, and 160 or more is evidence of distress. The real danger is when the rate is 20 beats slower than normal, and the rhythm possibly irregular also. (Normal rhythm is a short sound followed by a longer sound; each pair completes one pumping action of the heart muscle, and counts as one beat.) Occasionally beats may be missed altogether, and a count of 110 or less is cause for grave concern.

Anything causing a change in the mother's blood pressure upsets the baby's system. Check that she is not lying flat on her back, or has not been semi-reclining — as in the classical LaMaze position — for too long. In either instance, a change in her position (preferably have her lie on her side) will stabilise her blood pressure once more, and often the baby's heart rate returns to normal.

If you can discount these causes, and the fetal heart

continues to demonstrate distress, the cause may be beyond your control, and may not be diagnosible until after the baby is born. The likely causes are: cord compression, cord around the neck, short cord, undue or prolonged pressure on the baby's head, or early separation of the placenta (which would be accompanied by bright red bleeding). The best thing the mother can do is to breathe slowly and deeply to provide as much oxygen as possible to the baby. If birth is imminent, get the baby pushed out as promptly as possible. If it is not, get to the hospital right away.

Hyperactivity occurs when a child is severely distressed — it is possibly convulsing, definitely struggling for oxygen and fighting for its life.

Meconium in the amniotic water is significant as a distress sign in head presentations, but is to be expected in a breech delivery (of course it will only be seen after the membranes have ruptured). When a baby is under distress, his anal sphincter relaxes; but sometimes the distress is temporary and the reason undeterminable. The fetal heart rate may change a little after meconium is passed, and the important thing is whether or not it returns quickly to normal, showing that the distress has passed. If this happens, as is likely, remain alert, but continue the birthing at home. The baby's heart rate, its strength and rhythm, is your guide.

A faint heart sound with a normal rate probably means only that the baby has moved slightly making the heart harder to hear.

It is quite possible for a baby who shows signs of distress at some point, to be born fine and healthy, although, statistically, he has a greater chance of needing help. If there is meconium staining, make sure you suction the baby's nose and mouth thoroughly before he attempts to breathe, as meconoium aspirated into the lungs can cause respiratory distress after the birth.

There are other conditions, well documented in midwifery texts and best left there. The emphasis here is on a fit, well-nourished mother and baby, and the probability that without drugs and interferences and various other hang-ups, these problems will not enter the scene. Familiarise yourself with the text book information, but don't lose your perspective over the less likely, rather intimidating complications. Whether and when to seek help during labour depends largely on your ability to remain cool and assess things clearly, and on the degree of experience of those attending the birth. Don't mess around if you feel you are out of your depth, and don't hesitate to phone a medical or more experienced person for their advice.

DURING DELIVERY

Cord Around Baby's Neck After the head is born, you have to look and feel to determine whether or not the cord is around the baby's neck. If it is, pull on it gently. It may be loosely wound and you can either pull it over the baby's head, or push it back over the shoulders as the baby is born. If the cord is too tight, you must clamp it in *two* places, two inches apart, and cut the cord in between the clamps. The mother must pant or blow to prevent from pushing while this is being done. Then have her help get the baby out promptly, as his oxygen supply is now cut off and he must establish breathing on his own.

Membranes Intact Sometimes the baby is born with the membranes still intact. Pinch the membranes and snip them, then peel them away from the baby's face.

Knot in Cord Always handle the birth with gentle unhurried movements. This way, if there happens to be a loose knot in the cord (which does infrequently happen in early pregnancy during a playful somersault) you won't put sudden tension on it and tighten it. If the knot has pulled tight during the birth, you will be treating an asphyxiated baby. If it is possible to loosen the knot, do so.

Short Umbilical Cord   Two births that I know of personally have involved an unusually short umbilical cord — this is a rare occurence. In both instances, the baby was able to descend quite normally, but became distressed soon after the head became visible. Both mothers felt the sudden need to get the baby born right away and did so with a tremendous push which caused them to tear badly, but probably saved the babies' lives.

An extremely short cord will prevent the baby from moving down into the birth canal; fetal distress and failure of labour to progress will be your reasons for getting medical assistance.

Posterior Presentation   Occasionally a baby will not turn, but remains in this posterior position. He can he born this way, but it will be a harder labour for the mother and she will have to stretch more than usual, as a larger diameter of the baby's head presents. After the head is born, you may see it rotate 270 degrees instead of the usual 90.

Face Presentation   Sometimes too, the baby's head will not fully flex; depending on whether it is partially flexed or not at all, the baby will be born face or brow first. A face-first baby's head is fully extended, and from all the pressure on his face during labor, his face will be swollen and distorted and his voice hoarse. This looks more alarming than it actually is, and will quickly settle down. Face presentations occur only once in 500 births.

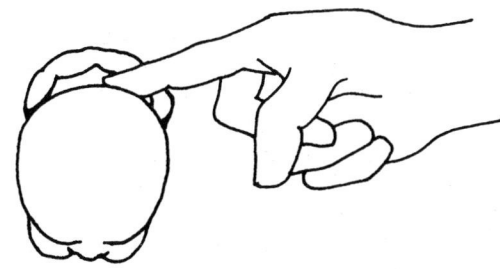

Fig.1

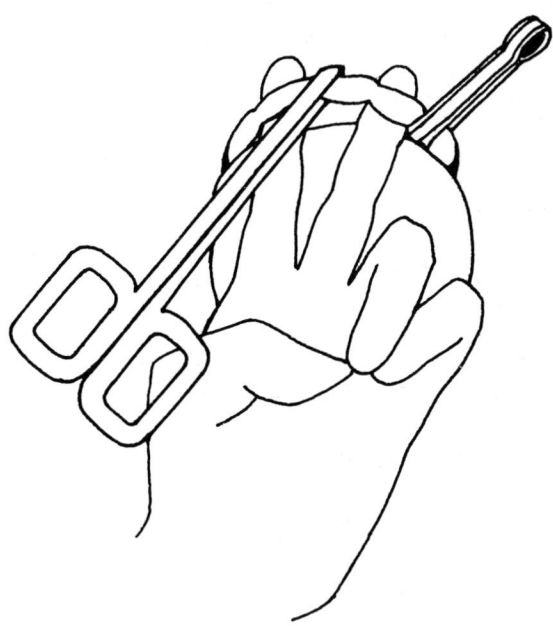

Fig.2

Cord Around Neck

Fig.1 Feeling for the cord.

Fig.2 Two methods of clamping the cord prior to cutting it between the clamps.

You should get help, if you don't have a midwife with you, once you realise it is a face presentation. The delivery is easier to manage if the chin can be born first; the facial bones do not overlap and thus a large, inflexible diameter is presenting. If the chin gets hung-up, an episiotomy (and sometimes forceps) would be required.

Moulding of the Fetal Head

These four diagrams show the moulding when baby was in:

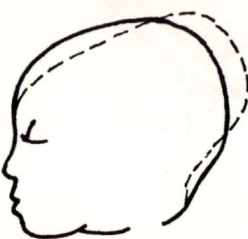

Fig.1 Anterior presentation

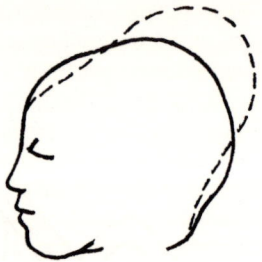

Fig.2 Posterior presentation

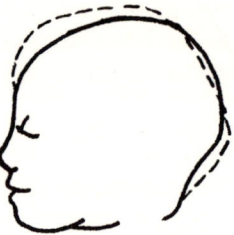

Fig.3 Brow presentation

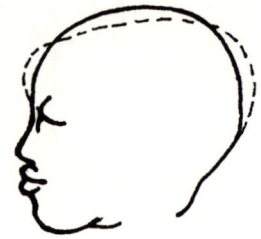

Fig.4 Face presentation

Brow Presentation   A brow presentation occurs when the baby's head is halfway between fully flexed and fully extended. Fortunately, it is a rare occurence — about one in every 2000 births — as a full term baby may not be able to be born vaginally. Most brow presentations occur in premature births and, as the baby is small, vaginal birth is possible. After such a birth, the baby's face is swollen and distorted and his brow temporarily discoloured.

The Asphyxiated Baby   A healthy baby will breathe within 30 to 60 seconds of birth. A mildly asphyxiated baby may be bluish, with weak muscle tone, may not cry, or may breathe irregularly. Do the APGAR assessment. If the pulse is above 100, there is no immediate danger, he justs needs gentle stimulation. Suction his nostrils, making sure his head is lower than the rest of his body so that fluids will drain out. If it seems necessary, wipe out the baby's mouth with a sterile gauze square. These babies respond well to touch. Gently stroke his spine, from the base upwards; stroke the soles of his feet; blow gently over his abdomen and chest. It is important to make him cry and expand his lungs well, then he will generally make a rapid recovery.

If the baby is limp and white or blue, with an APGAR score of 4 or less, he is severely asphyxiated, and will need resuscitation. Keep him warm while you carry this out, as chilling will endanger him more. When you resuscitate a baby, the aims are: to clear the air-passage, and to maintain both breathing and circulation.

Suction the baby to ensure all mucous is removed from his airway. If this does not stimulate him to breathe, begin resuscitation. If you are able to have an infant resuscitation bag mask for your birth, get familiar with how it works beforehand. Squeeze it at a rate of 24 puffs per minute. Mouth-to-mouth resuscitation accomplishes the same thing — it maintains breathing and supplies oxygen. Cover his face with a sterile gauze square, seal his nose and mouth with your mouth, lift his chin to straighten his air passage, and puff into him 24 times a minute. Baby lungs are very fragile and their capacity is small. When you learn resuscitation measures before the birth, practice puffing the small amounts of air needed to inflate their little lungs without damaging them — about one adult mouthful.

If the baby's heart rate is 60 or less, his circulation will be very poor. Cardiac massage should be combined with the mouth-to-mouth or infant-bag resuscitation. To perform cardiac massage, lie the baby on a firm surface, lay your thumbs on his breastbone and wrap your fingers around his back. With your thumbs, depress the breastbone about one inch (2 - 3cm) at the rate of two per second. Mouth-to-mouth breaths should be given after every four or five compressions, between compressions. Try not to interrupt their rhythm, and maintain these two measures evenly and smoothly until the baby's heartrate beats regularly at the normal speed, at which point the massage is discontinued, and the mouth-to-mouth stops when he is breathing alone. Obviously, this requires good coordination between two people with only on-the-spot practice being possible. A third person should be organising the move of the child to the hospital, in which eventuality, the resuscitation measures would be carried out continuously until medical aid takes over.

These measures are well-described in *Spiritual Midwifery*, revised edition. Gregory White, in *Emergency Childbirth* describes the chest-compression method of resuscitation. This is advisable if you are not confident about doing 'mouth-to-mouth'.

If your child has a heartbeat, he has a chance. The though of facing the unexpected arrival of a 'flat' baby at home is very scary. But it does have positive aspects too. For some adults, being able to turn the baby over to machines and supposedly competent professionals may be a relief; but it may not be the best thing for the baby. While he is alive he receives 'vibrations', and I believe that if he *can* survive, he will do so in response to the desperate outpouring of love, energy and sheer will for him to live which comes from his parents and everyone else involved in the birth. I wonder how many distressed babies retreat even further after a traumatic birth and the hostile reception of our impersonal, medical mechanics.

Along with our natural feelings of helplessness in such a crisis, we must remember too, the possible disasters of technology — all the people who must live subnormal lives because they were saved at birth, forced to live when nature would have conceded a merciful death.

Stillbirth When stillbirths occur, parents are much better able to cope with it at home. Parents who are able to hold and be with their child find it possible to later part with him and accept his death. It hurts, as badly as anything can hurt, but the experience remains positive and growthful. Feelings and emotions are not denied or shut away; the baby, carried for nine months and recently delivered is not immediately hidden away as if to deny that he ever existed. The parents can treat the child with the tenderness and respect they feel for him, even though his life is absent; grief is not immediately intruded on by social demands and hospital customs. We are finally becoming aware that privacy in those initial hours is most important to the grieving family.

Hospital-delivered mothers of stillborn children grieve a lot longer, and sometimes never work through the experience properly because of how the event is falsified by well-meaning but insensitive hospital and social policies. The mother-father-child relationship remains forever unconcluded and unresolvable.

The Farm Midwives have included stillbirth experiences in their book: *Christina's Birth and Burial*, is a particularly anguished, but meaningful, human story. There is also a special little book by William Kotzwinkle called *Swimmer in the Secret Sea*, a very tender story of birth and death (published by Avon

Books).

During pregnancy, I think it is natural, even compulsive at some point, to think about death. Doctors, and society in general, would rather we push these thoughts away, calling them ridiculous or paranoid. But allow yourself your thoughts, they are important. Part of taking responsibility for birth is working out how much you can take on. Presuming you, or one person present at the birth, will be fully versed in emergency measures, can you accept these limits of human resources? Can you accept that if these measures fail, the child was, for some reason, not meant to live? No matter where births take place, there will always be some infant deaths — that's a fact of life every pregnant couple must accept. Can you accept it in your home? You must recognise that society (as reflected by people holding high office) will not share your values, and may even want to incriminate you or your midwife. Lester Hazell points out that if a child dies in hospital, regardless of the cause of death, no-one is to blame, but if a child is born at home with a club foot, it is your fault!

Stillbirth at home is, statistically, a very rare event. As you think about it, keep in mind the added safety of unmedicated, unhurried, carefully-prepared-for homebirth. The parents who have taken all the physical, nutritional, and emotional precautions to provide their baby with the best possible reserves, should not allow themselves to feel guilt if the unexpected does happen.

AFTER THE BIRTH

Delayed Birth of the Placenta   After the baby is born, the uterine wall continues to contract and squeezes (separates) the placenta from it. This usually happens shortly, 10 to 20 minutes, after the birth. A hormone is responsible for this process, and it is released by the pituitary in response to the suckling stimulation of the baby. So when the baby is nursed soon after birth, difficulties with the third stage seldom occur.

If the placenta is not delivered after half an hour, have the woman squat; sometimes it has separated and is just sitting in the birth canal. If it still doesn't appear, give the baby every opportunity to suck strongly. If he is not too obliging, stimulate her nipples manually instead — it should work just as well.

Be familiar with the techniques for massaging the uterus to stimulate expulsive contractions. A small rush of dark blood usually indicates separation has occurred. During this stage it is still important not to hurry things and stay calm. A stubborn placenta may separate if the woman moves around a little. If there is no bleeding and she feels alright, there is no need to hurry the third stage, but if she is experiencing strong cramps, the placenta may have separated and be trapped in the contracting uterus. Encourage her to relax, even sleep, lying on her stomach. The placenta will probably slide out when she awakens and squats.

Some women have waited several hours for the placenta to emerge. Whether or not you decide to just sit it out depends on two conditions: there must be no bleeding, and the mother must feel fine. If either condition fails, get advice. NEVER become tempted to pull on the cord. Unnatural forced separation will almost always lead to excess bleeding; it will also be very painful, as is the rough abdominal prodding employed by some doctors.

Bleeding   As the placenta separates, a gush of blood will be noticed. After the placenta is born, about half a cup of blood loss is to be expected (if it is contained in a bowl it is much easier to estimate).

Beyond this, bleeding to worry about is bright, red blood running out in a steady stream. Have the mother lie down, and raise her pelvis on pillows; keep her comfortably warm and give her moral support while you gently massage the uterus, causing it to contract and close off the blood vessels. An ice-pack on her tummy is often effective in stopping bleeding.

In *Commonsense Childbirth*, Lester Hazell describes an English doctor who uses raw placenta to stop bleeding; her patients must eat a small portion — as is, or blended with tomato juice — and claims it works as soon as the placenta comes into contact with the mucous membrane of the mouth. She emphasises that it must be raw. (Maybe this explains why animals, who instinctively eat their placentas, do not seem prone to post-partum haemorrhages.) Also encourage the baby to nurse, or stimulate the nipples manually to produce natural contractions.

Try to establish the cause of the bleeding. The above measures will usually bring a slack uterus under control, although you must remain very wary and ready to repeat the procedures if it slackens up and bleeding resumes.

If a blood vessel has torn in a vaginal tear, you might have to get a stitch put in it to control bleeding from that source.

Check the placenta very carefully; if any has been retained in the uterus, it has to be removed by a doctor before bleeding will be controlled.

At the first sign of excess bleeding, the woman should be encouraged to eat the placenta — first a little raw, then the rest, quick-stewed or blended. Apart from its bleeding control properties, it has great revitalising power. It must be a fairly instinctive thing to do, for I've known strictly vegetarian women who have had a great urge to eat the placenta after their births, and thoroughly enjoyed it. After a haemorrhage, eating iron-rich foods is important to build up the blood and energy again. Do these things, get plenty of rest, and your recovery will not be greatly set back.

Shock   If excessive bleeding persists, the effects will be shown in the mother's appearance. She will gradually become more lethargic and pale, and display the following symptoms of shock: cold, clammy skin; lowered blood pressure; weak, thready pulse; shallower breathing; and eventually, a loss of consciousness.

Employ the following four measures promptly and you will likely stop the bleeding and revive the mother without having to get help.

1. Cover her to keep her warm; becoming either too cold or overheated will intensify her body distress.

2. Elevate her feet so that her blood circulation will concentrate around her vital organs.

3. Give her honey to eat; it enervates and strengthens the heart with a long-acting effect.

4. Get the woman to drink, quickly — all at once — a half glass of water into which one teaspoon of cayenne pepper has been stirred. Cayenne (red) pepper is enervating and will also help control bleeding. One could possibly prepare for this emergency beforehand by filling some gelatin capsules with cayenne. This measure, in particular, has often had immediate effect on both bleeding and shock, making medical assistance unnecessary.

(A "pill" of any herb can be made in the following manner: mix ground herb with honey to form a thick paste; drop a tablet-sized quantity onto a small piece of tissue paper; roll and twist ends. This is as easy to swallow, with water, as a gelatin capsule, and is an especially useful way to prepare herbs that are very bitter to the taste.)

Other useful herbs for all forms of shock are: leaves or fruit of the alder tree, clover blossoms — especially red clover, rosemary and skullcap. "Dr Bach's Shock Remedy" made from rock-rose is available in some health stores, and is most effective.

Perineal Tears   If a tear is more than half an inch long and you want an alternative to stitches, try this: grind or grate comfrey root (fresh or rehydrated) into a tacky pulp; hold the edges of the tear together and apply the pulp generously to cover the perineum. It will stick, and when dry it is hard, like a natural scab. The medicinal properties of comfrey will speed the natural healing.

— References —			
Positions of the Baby	**Midwifery**	**Page 58**	Diagrams
Mechanism of Labour	"	Page 59	"
Perineal Support	"	Page 66	"
Cord Around Neck	"	Page 67	"
Examination of Placenta	"	Page 32	"
Delivery of Placenta	**Rural Manual**	Page 50	"
	Spiritual Midwifery	Page 367	"
Emergency Resuscitation	**Emergency Childbirth** (descriptions)		
	Spiritual Midwifery, Revised Ed. (descriptions)		

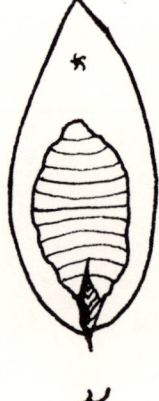

Fig.1

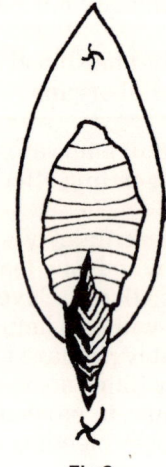

Fig.2

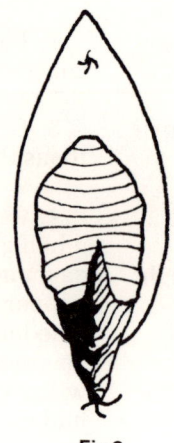

Fig.3

AFTER THE BIRTH

Perineal Tears

Fig.1 First degree tear — of thinned out skin and mucous membrane.

Fig.2 Second degree tear — extends into muscle tissue.

Fig.3 Third degree tear — the perineum has torn through to, and includes, the muscle sphincter of the anus.

— Reading —	
White, Gregory	Emergency Childbirth
Gaskin, Ina May	Spiritual Midwifery
Lang, Raven	Birth Book
Hallum, Jean	Midwifery
Hazell, Lester	Commonsense Childbirth

Pregnancy, Childbirth and the Newborn; a Manual for Rural Midwives.

Appendix II

SUPPLEMENTARY READING

The following books are especially recommended to supplement the information in this manual.

Immaculate Deception by Suzanne Arms, is a marvellous, comparative revelation of childbirth in America. I do not wish to go into a discussion of hospital practices and the evaluation of its technology in this manual designed for a natural homebirth, but some knowledge and understanding of them is an important part of your preparation, for several reasons: (1) you *may* have a hospital birth; distasteful as the idea might be, you owe it to yourself to be informed enough to make sound judgments should you unexpectedly need their services; (2) some prospective homebirth parents, in spite of their instincts, are unable to decide whether or not a birth at home is really safe without at least a few trimmings, like oxygen, pitocin, an I.V. perhaps. You need to understand all these measures, the reasons for their use in hospital, and the dangers associated with these measures; (3) if you don't have solid convictions for an alternative to hospital birth, this book will surely provide some!

Commonsense Childbirth by Lester Hazell is most enjoyable reading, offering a variety of important, useful information. She describes hospital practices and provides three comparative birth stories to evaluate their effects. Her attitude to birth is really good; her chapters describing labour, what happens and how it feels are perhaps the best in print. Equally reliable are the chapters on complications and what to do in various circumstances. A deeply sensitive chapter relates to tragedy and death.

Emergency Childbirth by Gregory White should be part of every birth kit, regardless of where birth is to take place. This brief manual will help you keep a sensible, natural perspective on birth; it outlines the basic procedures for birth and provides fingertip references for emergency situations.

Magical Child by Joseph Pearce, subtitled "Rediscovering Nature's Plan for our Children" is of lasting importance to every parent, and, through them, every child. Here is the most sensitive, understanding, brilliantly intuitive awareness of life, "... of any child entrusted to us — the offspring we begot or will beget, conceived or will conceive, and this child eternally begotten in ourselves". Here we are given a startling new insight into the growth, development and needs of the child from conception onwards. Those pregnant for the first time will feel relieved to have access to this fundamental knowledge 'in time'; while those who may have already suffered unhappy births, or gotten lost in the maze of unhelpful or confusing doctrines of childrearing will be reinforced as they realise the validity of their own gut instincts. We learn how our values and ideas interfere with the child's development, and how far-reaching are even minor interferences. A particularly valuable concept is Pearce's 'flow of reality' — from conception, the child is impressionable; gradually the impressions become discernible, and essential learning occurs in utero. Birth is a momentous, emotionally charged event; the needs of the minutes and hours after birth flow into the needs of the next years; at each moment, the experience is carried for a lifetime. Life is seen as a whole; birth is the neonatal beginning of the child's life, and perhaps the most significant peak in a woman's life cycle. When we get in touch with our babies before birth, then birth indeed becomes an exhilarating transition into physical and spiritual oneness with the child.

You will also need a Midwifery Text. There are several to choose from. I use, and have made specific reference to, the following books which I find easy to learn from and readily available:

Hallum, Jean.   **Midwifery**

Eloesser, Galt & Hemmingway
    Pregnancy, Childbirth and the Newborn : A Manual for Rural Midwives.
It is 'old-fashioned' in some ways, but very useful.
    Available by writing to:
        Institutio Indigestista Interamericano,
        Ninos, Heros, 139, Mexico 7, D.F.
    Specify English Edition; cost approx. $4.

You will also need a book on preparation for childbirth (and/or attend classes). Choose the method you feel suits you — see Chapter *Preparation for Labour*.

Bradley, Robert.   **Husband-Coached Childbirth**

Hathaway, Marjie & Jay   **Children at Birth**
    This is by two Bradley-method instructors — a marvellous book in many ways, especially the photographs.

Ewy, Donna & Roger   **Preparation for Childbirth. LaMaze**

Kitzinger, Sheila.   **The Experience of Childbirth**
    Presents the psychosexual method.

There are also several fine books on Homebirth:

Lang, Raven.   **Birth Book**

Hathaway, Marjie & Jay   **Children at Birth**

Sousa, Marion   **Childbirth at Home**

Bean, Constance   **Labour and Delivery: An Observer's Diary**
    This is valuable for its varying perspectives and evaluation of alternatives.

LeBoyer, Frederick.   **Birth Without Violence**
    I don't believe labour need be as frightening an experience as he supposes, but his sensitivity towards the child is special.

May, Ina. and the Farm Midwives   **Spiritual Midwifery**
    The revised edition contains a comprehensive and clearly presented section on midwifery; however, it does contain a few inaccuracies and should not be your only source of midwifery information. The birth stories are gem-like accounts of human experience, portraying spiritual and sexual aspects of birth which just a couple of generations of hospital birthing have obliterated. This book awakens our awareness and kindles enthusiasm for the learning we must do for a safe, spiritual birth.

A book on breastfeeding is most worthwhile:

Pryor, Karen.   **Nursing Your Baby**
    A proven classic.

Ewy, Donna & Roger   **Preparation for Breastfeeding**

Kipley, Sheila.   **Breastfeeding and Natural Child Spacing.**
    This is a favourite; its subtitle "The Ecology of Natural Mothering" describes it nicely.

If your local bookstores are not too well stocked, you can get these books from the International Childbirth Association. For their Book List, write to:

    Bookmarks,
    I.C.E.A. Book Centre,
    P.O. Box 20048,
    Minneapolis, Minn. 55420
        U.S.A.

You do not have to be a member. Their prices are regular List Prices and the selection is comprehensive. (Prompt delivery, too.)

Also check out for a Childbirth Education group in your area; they may have a small lending library. Even small public libraries are carrying more childbirth and parenting books nowadays.

APGAR Assessment

                                                              60 Sec.   5 Mins.

A - appearance (colour)
- 2 if the skin is completely pink ☐ ☐
- 1 if body is pink, and limbs or feet are bluish ☐ ☐
- 0 if entire body is blue ☐ ☐

P - pulse
- 2 if above 100 per minute ☐ ☐
- 1 if less than 100 per minute ☐ ☐
- 0 if pulse/heartbeat is absent ☐ ☐

G - grimace* (annoyed response to suctioning or stroking the sole of the foot)
- 2 if cries vigorously ☐ ☐
- 1 if grimaces or cries a little ☐ ☐
- 0 if no response ☐ ☐

A - activity*
- 2 if making active motions ☐ ☐
- 1 if some leg/arm movement ☐ ☐
- 0 if motionless and limp ☐ ☐

R - respiration (breathing)
- 2 if strong efforts to breathe ☐ ☐
- 1 if breathing slow and irregular ☐ ☐
- 0 if not breathing ☐ ☐

Baby's Name ....

Date ....

TOTALS: _____

*The baby may be quite relaxed after a calm birth; there will be no vigorous protests to calculate from, and no desire on your part to stimulate any. You can estimate these points by observing tentative, explorative movements the baby will make — even a relaxed baby makes involuntary unco-ordinated movements. If this is happening, you won't need to provoke the child, especially if the score for the other signs is good. In hospital, the baby is usually protesting a catheter stuck down his throat, a slap on the bottom, or being dangled by his ankles.

Apart from counting the pulse, the rest falls into your general appraisal of the child. Have an APGAR chart drawn up ahead of time and call out your scores to the person handling it. Here is a sample chart for easy use; just tick beside the appropriate description.

APGAR Assessment   60 Sec.   5 Mins.

A - appearance (colour)
- 2 if the skin is completely pink ☐ ☐
- 1 if body is pink, and limbs or feet are bluish ☐ ☐
- 0 if entire body is blue ☐ ☐

P - pulse
- 2 if above 100 per minute ☐ ☐
- 1 if less than 100 per minute ☐ ☐
- 0 if pulse/heartbeat is absent ☐ ☐

G - grimace* (annoyed response to suctioning or stroking the sole of the foot)
- 2 if cries vigorously ☐ ☐
- 1 if grimaces or cries a little ☐ ☐
- 0 if no response ☐ ☐

A - activity*
- 2 if making active motions ☐ ☐
- 1 if some leg/arm movement ☐ ☐
- 0 if motionless and limp ☐ ☐

R - respiration (breathing)
- 2 if strong efforts to breathe ☐ ☐
- 1 if breathing slow and irregular ☐ ☐
- 0 if not breathing ☐ ☐

Baby's Name ....

Date ....

TOTALS: _____ _____

*The baby may be quite relaxed after a calm birth; there will be no vigorous protests to calculate from, and no desire on your part to stimulate any. You can estimate these points by observing tentative, explorative movements the baby will make — even a relaxed baby makes involuntary unco-ordinated movements. If this is happening, you won't need to provoke the child, especially if the score for the other signs is good. In hospital, the baby is usually protesting a catheter stuck down his throat, a slap on the bottom, or being dangled by his ankles.

Apart from counting the pulse, the rest falls into your general appraisal of the child. Have an APGAR chart drawn up ahead of time and call out your scores to the person handling it. Here is a sample chart for easy use; just tick beside the appropriate description.

APGAR Assessment

		60 Sec.	5 Mins.

A - appearance (colour)
- 2 if the skin is completely pink ☐ ☐
- 1 if body is pink, and limbs or feet are bluish ☐ ☐
- 0 if entire body is blue ☐ ☐

P - pulse
- 2 if above 100 per minute ☐ ☐
- 1 if less than 100 per minute ☐ ☐
- 0 if pulse/heartbeat is absent ☐ ☐

G - grimace* (annoyed response to suctioning or stroking the sole of the foot)
- 2 if cries vigorously ☐ ☐
- 1 if grimaces or cries a little ☐ ☐
- 0 if no response ☐ ☐

A - activity*
- 2 if making active motions ☐ ☐
- 1 if some leg/arm movement ☐ ☐
- 0 if motionless and limp ☐ ☐

R - respiration (breathing)
- 2 if strong efforts to breathe ☐ ☐
- 1 if breathing slow and irregular ☐ ☐
- 0 if not breathing ☐ ☐

Baby's Name ....

Date ....

TOTALS: _____ _____

*The baby may be quite relaxed after a calm birth; there will be no vigorous protests to calculate from, and no desire on your part to stimulate any. You can estimate these points by observing tentative, explorative movements the baby will make — even a relaxed baby makes involuntary unco-ordinated movements. If this is happening, you won't need to provoke the child, especially if the score for the other signs is good. In hospital, the baby is usually protesting a catheter stuck down his throat, a slap on the bottom, or being dangled by his ankles.

Apart from counting the pulse, the rest falls into your general appraisal of the child. Have an APGAR chart drawn up ahead of time and call out your scores to the person handling it. Here is a sample chart for easy use; just tick beside the appropriate description.

APGAR Assessment

 60 Sec.   5 Mins.

A - appearance (colour)
- 2 if the skin is completely pink ☐ ☐
- 1 if body is pink, and limbs or feet are bluish ☐ ☐
- 0 if entire body is blue ☐ ☐

P - pulse
- 2 if above 100 per minute ☐ ☐
- 1 if less than 100 per minute ☐ ☐
- 0 if pulse/heartbeat is absent ☐ ☐

G - grimace* (annoyed response to suctioning or stroking the sole of the foot)
- 2 if cries vigorously ☐ ☐
- 1 if grimaces or cries a little ☐ ☐
- 0 if no response ☐ ☐

A - activity*
- 2 if making active motions ☐ ☐
- 1 if some leg/arm movement ☐ ☐
- 0 if motionless and limp ☐ ☐

R - respiration (breathing)
- 2 if strong efforts to breathe ☐ ☐
- 1 if breathing slow and irregular ☐ ☐
- 0 if not breathing ☐ ☐

Baby's Name ....

Date ....

TOTALS: _____   _____

*The baby may be quite relaxed after a calm birth; there will be no vigorous protests to calculate from, and no desire on your part to stimulate any. You can estimate these points by observing tentative, explorative movements the baby will make — even a relaxed baby makes involuntary unco-ordinated movements. If this is happening, you won't need to provoke the child, especially if the score for the other signs is good. In hospital, the baby is usually protesting a catheter stuck down his throat, a slap on the bottom, or being dangled by his ankles.

Apart from counting the pulse, the rest falls into your general appraisal of the child. Have an APGAR chart drawn up ahead of time and call out your scores to the person handling it. Here is a sample chart for easy use; just tick beside the appropriate description.